Doctors

Lab Literacy
for Canadian
Doctors

*A guide to ordering
the right tests for
better patient care*

Christopher Naugler, MD, MSc, editor

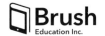

Brush Education Inc.
www.brusheducation.ca
contact@brusheducation.ca

Printed and manufactured in Canada
Ebook edition available at Amazon, Kobo, and other e-retailers.

Library and Archives Canada Cataloguing in Publication
Lab literacy for Canadian doctors: a guide to ordering the right
tests for better patient care / Christopher Naugler, MD, MSc.,
editor.
Includes indexes.
Issued in print and electronic formats.

ISBN 978-1-55059-491-1 (pbk.).—ISBN 978-1-55059-492-8
(epub).—ISBN 978-1-55059-493-5 (pdf).—ISBN 978-1-55059-
494-2 (mobi)

1. Diagnosis, Laboratory—Canada—Handbooks, manuals, etc.

I. Naugler, Christopher T. (Christopher Terrance), 1967–, editor
of compilation II. Title.

RB38.2.L33 2013   616.07'5 C2013-905642-4   C2013-905643-2

Produced with the assistance of the Government of Alberta,
Alberta Media Fund. We also acknowledge the financial support
of the Government of Canada through the Canada Book Fund for
our publishing activities.

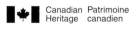

**Government
of Alberta** ■   Canadian Patrimoine
                     Heritage   canadien

Contents

Illustrations

Introduction

Why this guide?

Five years ago, new evidence about vitamin D alerted doctors to the impacts of vitamin D deficits on patient health. This drove a meteoric increase in vitamin D testing in labs across North America. At some clinics, vitamin D testing became one of the single biggest expenses in the budget for lab services.

For all those tests and all that money, you would expect that doctors were at least getting useful information from the results. But they weren't.

Vitamin D levels are not good predictors of bone health—or other health outcomes for that matter. Patients have different underlying disease susceptibilities, and, depending on supplements, their serum vitamin D levels go up and down. So, knowing a patient's current vitamin D level has dubious value.

Ample evidence, however, shows the benefits of vitamin D supplements for almost everyone, regardless of their baseline vitamin D level. Therefore, a strategy of "treat don't test" makes eminent sense and saves valuable health-care resources for testing that actually has a clinical impact.

In the setting of finite health-care resources, tradeoffs such as this—between clinical utility and costs of testing—will become increasingly important.

As health practitioners, we share an ethical responsibility to provide good stewardship of limited health-care dollars and testing resources. Whether you are a primary-care physician or resident, a medical student, or a health professional in an allied field, you need to be lab literate: you need to know which tests have the highest yield for the clinical situations you typically encounter.

Many references help you interpret lab investigations, but they don't tell you what investigations to do in the first place.

This guide is about what lab investigations to do *first*. We outline the most efficient and cost-effective way for you to use laboratory investigations to support clinical diagnosis and management.

How to use this guide

THE MAIN GUIDE

The guide is organized the way clinicians think: by clinical presentation and by organ system. So, if you have a patient with a skin problem, go to the section on dermatology. If a patient presents with fatigue, go to the section on fatigue.

In addition to information on lab investigations, we provide, where useful, differential diagnoses, etiologies, and summaries of signs and symptoms. We also share some "pearls"—particular knowledge about lab investigations we have gathered as experts and clinicians in our fields.

LAB BASICS

Lab investigations are only as good as the specimens delivered for analysis, and lab results are only as useful as human slip-ups and margins of error allow.

Find advice and information here on lab errors, false positives and negatives, and blood and tissue collection.

LAB INVESTIGATIONS INDEX

This index describes the diagnostic purpose of the lab investigations discussed in the guide, plus other common lab tests.

If you need a quick check on what an investigation is for, look it up here.

WHAT'S NOT IN THIS GUIDE

This guide focuses on laboratory investigations. It does not cover diagnostic imaging.

It covers typical disorders and clinical presentations. It does not cover every disorder and clinical presentation, and is not meant to replace sound clinical judgement.

A NOTE ABOUT UNITS

This guide gives laboratory values in both SI units (the International System of Units) and conventional units. We give the SI units first and the conventional units second.

We did this because Canadian laboratories generally, but not always, report test results in SI units. In addition, Canadian laboratories refer some esoteric tests to the United States, and laboratories in the United States generally, but again not always, report results in conventional units.

For these reasons, we felt it was important to provide laboratory values in both systems as a reference.

DISCLAIMER

The publishers, authors, contributors, and editors bring substantial expertise to this reference and have made their best efforts to ensure that it is useful, accurate, safe, and reliable.

Nonetheless, practitioners must always rely on their own experience, knowledge, and judgement when consulting any of the information contained in this reference or employing it in patient care. When using any of this information, they should remain conscious of their responsibility for their own safety and the safety of others, and for the best interests of those in their care.

To the fullest extent of the law, neither the publishers, the authors, the contributors, nor the editors assume any liability for injury or damage to persons or property from any use of information or ideas contained in this reference.

Dermatology

Dr. Ethan Flynn

ABBREVIATIONS

ALC-1	anti–liver cytosol antibody type 1	FTA-ABS	fluorescent treponemal antibody absorption test
ALKM-1	anti–liver kidney microsomal antibody type 1	GGT	γ-glutamyltransferase
ALP	alkaline phosphatase	HSV	herpes simplex virus
ALT	alanine aminotransferase	ICE	immune-capture EIA
AMA	antimitochondrial antibodies	IFA	immunofluorescent assay
ANA	antinuclear antibody	IgA	immunoglobulin A
anti-TPO	anti–thyroid peroxidase	IgG	immunoglobulin G
ASMA	anti–smooth muscle antibody	IgM	immunoglobulin M
AST	aspartate aminotransferase	KOH	potassium hydroxide
BUN	blood urea nitrogen	LCR	ligase chain reaction
CBC	complete blood count	MHA-TP	microhemagglutination assay–*Treponema pallidum*
CRP	C-reactive protein		
CSF	cerebrospinal fluid	MRSA	methicillin-resistant *Staphylococcus aureus*
DFA	direct fluorescence assay		
DIC	disseminated intravascular coagulation	NAAT	nucleic acid amplification testing
		PCR	polymerase chain reaction
eGFR	estimated glomerular filtration rate	PT/INR	prothrombin time or international normalized ratio
EIA	enzyme immunoassay	RPR	rapid plasma reagin
ELISA	enzyme-linked immunosorbent assay	RT-PCR	reverse transcription polymerase chain reaction
ESR	erythrocyte sedimentation rate		

SSSS	staphylococcal scalded skin syndrome	TSH	thyroid-stimulating hormone (thyrotropin)
STD	sexually transmitted disease	tTG	tissue transglutaminase
T_4	thyroxine	TTP	thrombotic thrombocytopenic purpura
TPPA	*Treponema pallidum* particle agglutination	VDRL	Venereal Disease Research Laboratory test

OVERALL APPROACH

Key steps in diagnosis

The correct algorithm for proper skin pathology diagnosis depends on:

- a thorough clinical history
- a complete physical exam (including mucous membranes)

Before pursuing any laboratory tests, the clinician should determine whether a disorder is:

- primary (a disease arising from, and typically localized to, the skin): for these disorders, clinical laboratory tests typically have dubious utility
- a cutaneous manifestation of a systemic disease: when systemic disease is suspected or cannot be ruled out, laboratory testing of serum, plasma, or even urine is useful

Diagnosis of primary skin disease may also require:

- tissue biopsy with histopathological evaluation
- Tzanck smear, in which the exfoliated squamous cells of an unroofed vesicle are evaluated microscopically for viral cytopathic morphologic changes

Radiologic evaluation may occasionally be used, mostly in metastatic neoplastic or paraneoplastic etiologies of cutaneous disease.

SKIN BIOPSY PROCEDURES

CHOOSING THE RIGHT PROCEDURE

Skin biopsy involves a minor surgical procedure.

- Specimens should generally sample both the lesion and adjacent nonlesional skin.
- If the margin of a lesion is not well defined, sample lesional and nonlesional skin (as clinically indicated) with separate specimens.
- If possible, sample untraumatized skin (e.g., not scratched); this is particularly an issue with itchy skin rashes.

Determine what biopsy procedure to use based on the clinical presentation of a cutaneous lesion, in particular its depth (see the breakdown that follows).

Biopsy procedure	When to use
Excisional biopsy	Pigmented skin lesions
	Clinically worrisome primary cutaneous neoplasms
	Histologically confirmed carcinoma (e.g., basal cell carcinoma): perform a complete excision
Punch biopsy	Cutaneous processes with suspected involvement of the dermis (e.g., nonneoplastic, inflammatory dermatoses)
	• punch biopsies provide a representative sample of the epidermis and full-thickness dermis
	• larger punch biopsies also provide subcutaneous fat, which is important in the evaluation of panniculitides (inflammatory conditions of the pannus)
Shave biopsy	Conditions involving or arising from the epidermis (useful for primary diagnosis of suspected skin cancer, with excision following histologic confirmation)

FIXED VERSUS FRESH SPECIMENS

The vast majority of biopsy specimens are fixed in formalin (10% aqueous formaldehyde).

In addition to formalin-fixed specimens, fresh specimens are useful for some conditions, including:

- infectious dermatitis
- suspected primary cutaneous lymphoproliferative neoplasms (such as cutaneous T-cell lymphoma)
- vesiculobullous dermatoses
- vasculitides

Submit fresh skin specimens to the laboratory moist in saline gauze.

Note that microbiologic culture studies or flow cytometry studies for lymphoma evaluation cannot be performed on formalin-fixed or alcohol-fixed tissue specimens.

DISORDERS AND CLINICAL PRESENTATIONS

"BUMPS" ON SKIN

KEYS TO WORKUP

Definitive diagnosis of "bumps" on the skin frequently rests on histopathologic evaluation of a punch or shave biopsy.

Note that cutaneous "bumps" may occasionally signal:

- subcutaneous pathologic conditions (e.g., soft tissue tumours or lymphadenopathy), for which biopsy and histopathologic diagnosis may be required
- developmental abnormalities or cutaneous manifestations of malignancy in infants[1]

LAB INVESTIGATIONS

SKIN BIOPSY

The vast majority of "bumps" are primary skin conditions, usually diagnosed by clinical impression along with skin biopsy and histopathologic evaluation.

MICROBIOLOGIC OR PROVIDER-PERFORMED STUDIES

In cases of suspected or presumed infectious dermatitides presenting as "bumps," the following tests can be useful:

- skin bacterial culture
- KOH scrape prep wet mount evaluation (for suspected fungal dermatitis)

DEPIGMENTATION

KEYS TO WORKUP

Depigmentation may be partial (such as following trauma) or complete (such as vitiligo).

Causes of depigmentation include:

- infection (especially fungal)
- dermatitis
- trauma
- exogenous steroid-associated causes
- albinism

LAB INVESTIGATIONS

PROVIDER-PERFORMED MICROSCOPY FOR WET MOUNT KOH PREP

Use as clinically indicated.

SKIN BIOPSY WITH HISTOPATHOLOGIC EVALUATION

Use as clinically indicated.

DRY SKIN

KEYS TO WORKUP

Dry skin is a common clinical symptom and may be associated with a wide array of factors and conditions, including:

- harsh soaps
- pools or hot tubs with heavy chlorination
- malnutrition
- hypothyroidism
- Addison syndrome
- vitamin A deficiency
- seasonal factors
- side effects of medications
- dry environment
- aging
- frequent bathing or bathing in hot water
- harsh scrubbing of skin
- contact dermatitis
- lichen simplex chronicus

Laboratory testing may be helpful in cases where a thorough investigation into clinical history (e.g., frequent use of harsh soaps, swimming in chlorinated water, frequent hot tub use, etc.) fails to elucidate a cause.

LAB INVESTIGATIONS

SKIN BIOPSY

This may be helpful in diagnosing contact dermatitis and lichen simplex chronicus.

Only use skin biopsy after ruling out environmental and nutritional factors (see the list under "keys to workup").

TESTS FOR HYPOTHYROIDISM

If clinical findings suggest hypothyroidism:

- Start by measuring thyroid-stimulating hormone (TSH), which is the single best initial test for thyroid disorders.
- Follow up with a repeat TSH plus a T_4 if the initial TSH is elevated.

See: hypothyroidism, p. 37

TESTS FOR ADRENAL INSUFFICIENCY (RARE)

Depending on clinical findings, test for adrenal insufficiency (Addison syndrome).

See: adrenal insufficiency, p. 24

HAIR LOSS

KEYS TO WORKUP

Alopecia, or hair loss, may be:

- primary (a number of syndromes)
- secondary to medications, radiation therapy, or chemotherapy

Etiology of alopecia may be determined from clinical history and, where applicable, through punch biopsy and histopathology.

LAB INVESTIGATIONS

PUNCH BIOPSY

Typically, biopsies obtain separate specimens of normal and affected scalp for comparison.

PALE SKIN

KEYS TO WORKUP

Pale skin may result from vascular disease, coagulopathy, anemia, neurologic-mediated causes, medication-related causes, environmental causes, toxicologic causes, or nutritional causes.

Lab tests are useful in diagnosing only some causes of pale skin, including:

- autoimmune hemolytic anemia
- anemia due to other causes
- bleeding
- chemical poisoning
- DIC
- folate deficiency (rare in North America)
- malnutrition
- respiratory failure
- TTP
- vitamin B_{12} deficiency

LAB INVESTIGATIONS
Correlate patient history and physical findings to select appropriate laboratory testing.

Possible investigations include:

- tests for TTP or unexplained bleeding (*see: bleeding and bruising, p. 141*)
- serum chemistries (BUN, creatinine, electrolytes, glucose) to evaluate for metabolic or renal abnormalities
- tests to evaluate for malnutrition: albumin, prealbumin, and total protein
- tests for anemia (*see: anemia, p. 134*)

PIGMENTED LESIONS ON SKIN

KEYS TO WORKUP
For the management of melanoma, use the latest clinical practice guidelines.

If in doubt of the significance of a histologic interpretation or appropriate management, a call to the reporting pathologist is often the easiest way to determine further management.

LAB INVESTIGATIONS

EXCISIONAL BIOPSY

Place specimen in 10% formalin and order a pathology consultation.

PEARLS

Punch biopsies are not suitable for the evaluation of clinically worrisome pigmented lesions. In such cases, an excisional biopsy should always be performed if clinically feasible. Location and clinical history are key components in the evaluation of pigmented lesions.

Note that widespread differences exist in the interpretation and reporting of dysplastic (Clark) nevi. Melanocytic nevi reported as containing moderate to severe dysplasia or atypia should be removed in their entirety for histologic examination. Management of melanoma should be based on the latest clinical practice guidelines.

PRURITUS

KEYS TO WORKUP

Causes of chronic pruritus include:

- primary dermatologic (e.g., chicken pox, hives)
- systemic (cholestasis, chronic kidney disease, myeloproliferative disorders, hyperthyroidism)
- neuropathic
- psychogenic

The most common cause of itchy skin without rash is dry skin (xerosis). Dry skin can arise from excessive bathing or washing, prolonged use of heating or air conditioning, or hot or mild weather with low humidity.

Primary skin conditions causing itchiness usually occur in specific areas and are typically associated with bumps, blisters, or red, irritated skin. Diagnosis is primarily clinical; history of medication use is extremely important to rule out medication-associated pruritus.

Laboratory investigations are primarily useful in the following contexts:

- investigating systemic causes of pruritus (see Table 1)
- when the cause of pruritus is not apparent by clinical history and physical examination
- when laboratory findings are necessary to confirm a suspected disorder

Internal diseases causing itchiness usually affect the whole body. Except for excoriated areas, skin that is itchy from internal disease may look entirely normal.

Table 1. Examples of systemic disease causing pruritus

Disease	Lab investigations
Celiac disease	IgA tTG antibody (tTG)
	IgA antiendomysial antibody (EMA)
	Total IgA level
	See: celiac disease serologies, pp. 65–67
Diabetes mellitus	*See: diabetes, p. 27*
Hematologic malignancies or disorders – leukemia, lymphoma, myelodysplastic syndromes	*See: hematology, p. 133*
Hyperthyroidism	*See: hyperthyroidism, p. 33*
Iron deficiency anemia	*See: anemia, p. 134*
Kidney failure	Creatinine/eGFR
Liver disease	Albumin
	Ammonia
	Glucose
	Liver function tests: ALP, ALT, GGT (and, as indicated, AST, direct and indirect bilirubin, PT/INR)

Continued on p. 11

Continued from p. 10

Disease	Lab investigations

	If liver function tests are elevated, consider:
	• Viral hepatitis panel (*see pp. 71–72*)
	• Autoimmune hepatitis panel
	   ◦ immunoglobulins (total or IgG fraction typically elevated 1.5 X above normal in autoimmune hepatitis)
	   ◦ ASMA
	   ◦ anti-LKM-1
	   ◦ ALC-1
	   ◦ ANA
	   ◦ AMA

Shingles (herpes zoster)	Depending on local availability, order 1 of the following tests: • direct fluorescent antibody assay • PCR assay of vesicular fluid (to detect varicella zoster virus DNA)

LAB INVESTIGATIONS

TESTS FOR CHICKENPOX OR HSV

Note that chickenpox and herpes simplex virus (HSV) are usually clinically diagnosed.

For problematic cases, and depending on availability, order 1 of the following tests:

- Tzanck smear
- serologic testing
- vesicular fluid culture

TESTS FOR HIVES

In acute cases, laboratory studies are not indicated.

In chronic cases, consider:

- CBC, to check for elevated eosinophil count
- hepatitis B and C serology
- cryoglobulin and complement levels, if cryoglobulinemia is suspected

- TSH and anti-TPO, if hypothyroidism with or without Hashimoto thyroiditis is suspected
- ANA; ESR or CRP, if urticarial vasculitis or rheumatologic disorder is suspected

RASH

KEYS TO WORKUP

A detailed review of the diagnosis of rash based on clinical history and physical examination is beyond the scope of this guide.

Causes of rash are numerous: laboratory tests are occasionally of importance in arriving at a diagnosis or etiology, particularly when the rash represents a cutaneous manifestation of a systemic disease (see Table 2).

Table 2. Causes of rash for which lab tests may be useful

Type of rash	Causes
Bacterial	Impetigo
	Meningococcal infection
	Lyme disease
	Hidradenitis suppurativa
	Staphylococcal scalded skin syndrome (SSSS)
	Typhus
	Rocky Mountain spotted fever
	Folliculitis, bacterial
	Other bacterial infection (esp. *Staphylococcus, Streptococcus*)
	Acne
	MRSA
	Sexually transmitted diseases
	Scarlet fever
	Toxic shock syndrome
	Bacteria-associated erythema multiforme

Continued on p. 13

Continued from p. 12

Type of rash	Causes
Fungal	Folliculitis, fungal
	Ringworm (dermatophytosis)
	Tinea versicolor
	Intertrigo (*Candida*)
	Jock itch (tinea cruris)
Noninfectious	Rheumatoid arthritis
	Lupus
	Henoch-Schönlein purpura
Viral	Smallpox
	Molluscum contagiosum
	Chickenpox (varicella)
	Hand foot and mouth disease (coxsackievirus)
	Dengue fever
	Shingles (herpes zoster)
	Fifth disease (erythrovirus)
	Measles
	Monkeypox
	Roseola
	Herpangina (coxsackievirus)

Punch biopsy and histopathologic evaluation are critical in many cases of rash if the cause is not apparent from clinical history and physical examination.

Cultures of skin lesions and exudates can aid diagnosis of some infection-related rashes:

- cultures useful: if the rash is a nidus of the infection itself (as in impetigo or bacterial folliculitis)
- cultures not useful: if the rash is a pathophysiologic or inflammatory response to infection (such as petechiae from disseminated meningococcal infection, or erythema migrans rash of Lyme disease)

Lab tests should be tailored to the clinical severity of the presentation. For example, an otherwise healthy patient with impetigo does not require lab tests. By contrast, a patient presenting with septic shock and rash may require a wide array of tests.

WHEN TO START TREATMENT

Treat promptly if clinical findings point to infectious disease! Do not wait for lab results, which may take a week or longer, particularly with serology or reference lab send-outs. Delaying treatment may result in multisystem organ dysfunction or failure. Antibiotics may be changed or discontinued later based on culture and sensitivity results, results of other lab testing (see "lab investigations," which follows), and ongoing clinical impression.

LAB INVESTIGATIONS: INFECTION-ASSOCIATED RASHES

INITIAL TESTS

The recommended panel of initial tests for most infection-associated rashes includes:

- CBC
- serum chemistries: BUN, creatinine, electrolytes, glucose
- ESR or CRP
- urinalysis
- liver function tests: ALP, ALT, GGT (and, as indicated, AST, direct and indirect bilirubin, PT/INR)
- blood cultures

ABOUT SEROLOGY AND LYME DISEASE

Serologic testing is not helpful (and may be misleading) in early Lyme disease due to false-negative serology.

False-positive anti-*Borrelia* serology may possibly occur in conditions not associated with Lyme disease (e.g., babesiosis, ehrlichiosis, acrodermatitis chronica atrophicans). Consult the laboratory on potential cross-reactivity of the serologic test.

Serology can confirm a diagnosis of suspected Lyme disease as a follow-up **after** beginning immediate antibiotic therapy. Do not wait for laboratory results to begin treatment if clinical features are consistent with Lyme disease.[2]

Acute and convalescent-phase serologic testing has no role in determining efficacy of treatment for Lyme disease. Serology remains positive long after clinical resolution of the disease.

BACTERIAL CULTURE OF SKIN EXUDATE OR LESION

Based on clinical findings, use bacterial cultures to identify:

- toxic shock syndrome (*S. aureus*, group A *Streptococcus*)
- impetigo: if associated with postinfectious glomerulonephritis or if MRSA is suspected
- hidradenitis suppurativa (flares may be associated with bacterial superinfection)
- SSSS (may be culture-negative; PCR for toxin is available if clinically suspected)
- acne: only in treatment-refractory cases to rule out gram-negative folliculitis

ABOUT RESULTS FROM BACTERIAL CULTURES

The results of bacterial cultures may be negative, particularly in patients recently or concurrently treated with antibiotics.

Consider blood cultures if bacteremia seems likely, based on clinical findings—e.g., low likelihood in cellulitis (2%), high likelihood in septic shock

(69%). Note that isolated leukocytosis and isolated elevation in temperature, in and of themselves, are poor predictors of bacteremia, unless clinical findings suggest an immunocompromised state or bacterial endocarditis.[3]

Many bacteria are difficult to grow in culture: be aware of alternative tests (such as serology or PCR), and beware of excluding a clinically suspected disease based on negative-culture results.

TESTS FOR SPECIFIC INFECTIONS
Test for specific infections based on clinical evidence (see the breakdown that follows).

Infection	Tests
Chickenpox (varicella zoster virus)	Tzanck smear of skin lesion for cytologic evaluation
	Serologic testing for varicella zoster virus
	Viral culture of skin lesion fluid
Coxsackievirus-associated mucocutaneous rash (hand-foot-and-mouth disease, herpangina)	Viral culture
	Immunoassay
	Serologic testing (acute and convalescent)
	PCR
	Vesicle fluid (if available) swab, and rectum or pharynx swab
Dengue fever (*Flavivirus*)	Viral culture (serum, plasma, leukocytes)
	IgG or IgM antibodies: diagnostic results show a 4-fold or greater rise in sequential titres in antibodies to 1 or more dengue antigens
	PCR of dengue-associated DNA (serum or CSF)
Measles	Serologic testing for IgG and IgM antibodies
– typically diagnosed clinically: use lab tests to confirm problematic cases	Viral culture
	RT-PCR (when available)

Continued on p. 17

Continued from p. 16

Infection	Tests
Rickettsial disease (typhus, Rocky Mountain spotted fever)	EIA or IFA to evaluate: • rise in IgM titre (acute primary disease) • rise in IgG titre (secondary immune response) PCR of skin or blood sample Latex agglutination Complement fixation (CF) test
Rickettsia-like disease (anaplasmosis, ehrlichiosis)	Evaluation of buffy coat preparation for WBC intracellular morulae Anti-*Anaplasma* or anti-*Ehrlichia* IgG (EIA, IFA) Acute and convalescent antibody titres (EIA, IFA)
Scarlet fever	Throat culture Blood culture Rapid streptococcal serum test (antideoxyribonuclease B or antistreptolysin O titre)
STDs	
• chlamydia	Midstream or first-void urine for nucleic acid amplification testing (NAAT) Urethral, oral, genital, anal swabs (as clinically indicated) for culture, DFA, ELISA or EIA, NAAT, DNA probe
• gonorrhea	Urethral, oral, genital, anal swabs (as clinically indicated) for culture, DNA probe, PCR, LCR
• syphilis – traditional screening method	Testing algorithm: • Begin with RPR • If RPR is positive, use a treponemal assay for confirmation: VDRL, FTA-ABS, MHA-TP, TPPA, or ICE syphilis recombinant antigen test (new, not widely available) • If RPR and the first treponemal assay are discordant (i.e., RPR positive, treponemal assay negative), order a second treponemal assay
• syphilis – reverse screening algorithm (gaining wider acceptance because the initial screening test is an automated EIA test, not a manual test)	Testing algorithm: • Begin with VDRL, FTA-ABS, or MHA-TP • If the initial test is positive, order RPR • If the initial test is positive and RPR is negative, order TPPA[4]

LAB INVESTIGATIONS: RASHES NOT ASSOCIATED WITH INFECTION

PUNCH BIOPSY

Biopsy is frequently helpful when clinical findings do not point to a clear cause of noninfectious rash.

BLOOD TESTS

Blood tests are generally less helpful than biopsy.

The exceptions are rashes associated with systemic illness, including:

- rash as a paraneoplastic syndrome or pathophysiologic sequela of malignancy
- rash as a cutaneous manifestation of systemic vasculitic illness (purpura or petechiae)
- rash associated with autoimmune disease, such as lupus

In these cases, blood tests should be directed toward the suspected systemic illness.

REFERENCES

1 Farvolden D, Sweeney SM, Wiss K. Lumps and bumps in neonates and infants. *Dermatol Ther*. 2005;18(2):104–116. http://dx.doi.org/10.1111/j.1529-8019.2005.05016.x. Medline:15953140

2 Potok OV, Brassard A. Lyme borreliosis: an update for Canadian dermatologists. *J Cutan Med Surg*. 2013;17(1):13–21. Medline:23364145

3 Coburn B, Morris AM, Tomlinson G, et al. Does this adult patient with suspected bacteremia require blood cultures? *JAMA*. 2012;308(5):502–511. http://dx.doi.org/10.1001/jama.2012.8262. Medline:22851117

4 Centers for Disease Control and Prevention (CDC). Discordant results from reverse sequence syphilis screening—five laboratories, United States, 2006–2010. *MMWR Morb Mortal Wkly Rep*. 2011;60(5):133–137. Medline:21307823

Ears, nose, and throat, and respiratory system

Dr. Christopher Naugler

ABBREVIATIONS

COPD   chronic obstructive pulmonary disease

OVERALL APPROACH

The diagnosis of most ear, nose, and throat ailments, and respiratory ailments, comes from a careful history and physical examination.

Most presentations do not require laboratory testing.

DISORDERS AND CLINICAL PRESENTATIONS

ASTHMA

KEYS TO WORKUP
Diagnosis is based on the presence of compatible signs and symptoms, family history, pulmonary function testing, and response to treatment.

LAB INVESTIGATIONS
Routine investigations are not recommended.

PEARLS

Asthmatic individuals may have an elevated IgE, but this test is not useful in establishing a diagnosis. Serum allergy testing is generally not useful, either: it delivers results with high false-positive and false-negative rates.

COUGH, ACUTE

KEYS TO WORKUP

Findings from patient history and physical exam should guide decisions about testing.

In the vast majority of cases, lab tests are not indicated.

The exception is if you suspect a cough arises from another medical condition, such as heart disease. Base your decision about lab tests on their utility for diagnosing the suspected underlying disease. The key is to rule out life-threatening conditions (e.g., pneumonia, exacerbation of severe asthma or COPD, pulmonary embolus, heart failure).

LAB INVESTIGATIONS

Routine investigations are not recommended.

OTITIS MEDIA, ACUTE

KEYS TO WORKUP

Diagnosis is clinical, based on the presence of compatible signs and symptoms.

LAB INVESTIGATIONS

Routine investigations are not recommended.

RHINOSINUSITIS

KEYS TO WORKUP

Diagnosis of acute bacterial rhinosinusitis is clinical, based on the presence of compatible signs and symptoms lasting more than 7 days.

LAB INVESTIGATIONS
Routine investigations are not recommended.

PEARLS
Routine nasal culture is not recommended.

If culture becomes necessary due to complications, obtain a specimen through maxillary tap or endoscopy.

SORE THROAT, ACUTE

KEYS TO WORKUP
Diagnosis is clinical, based on the presence of compatible signs and symptoms.

Clinical scoring systems stratify patient risk for group A streptococcal infection (e.g., Centor score, McIsaac score). In the McIsaac score,[1] each of the following scores a point:

- temperature higher than 38°C (100.4°F)
- absence of cough
- tender anterior cervical adenopathy
- tonsillar swelling or exudate
- patient age between 3 and 14 years

Subtract a point for patients aged 45 years or older.

LAB INVESTIGATIONS

THROAT CULTURE
Order this if a patient:

- has a score of 2 or 3; initiate treatment if the culture is positive
- has a score of 4; culture and initiate treatment simultaneously

For patients with a score of 0 or 1, routine throat culture is generally not necessary.

RAPID ANTIGEN TEST
This test has the advantage of providing a rapid answer, and most commercial kits have sensitivities

in the range of 90% and specificities in the range of 95%.

The rapid antigen test is offered by some labs and also as a point-of-care test for office uses.

PEARLS

A negative rapid antigen test does not need follow-up with a throat culture or tests for inflammatory markers.

REFERENCES

1   McIsaac WJ, White D, Tannenbaum D, et al. A clinical score to reduce unnecessary antibiotic use in patients with sore throat. *CMAJ*. 1998;158(1):75–83. Medline:9475915

FURTHER READING

Becker A, Lemière C, Bérubé D, et al. Asthma guidelines working group of the Canadian Network for Asthma Care: summary of recommendations from the Canadian Asthma Consensus guidelines, 2003. *CMAJ*. 2005;173(6 suppl):S3–11. Medline:16157733

Desrosiers M, Evans GA, Keith PK, et al. Canadian clinical practice guidelines for acute and chronic rhinosinusitis. *Allergy Asthma Clin Immunol*. 2011;7(1):2. http://dx.doi.org/10.1186/1710-1492-7-2. Medline:21310056

Dicpinigaitis PV, Colice GL, Goolsby MJ, et al. Acute cough: a diagnostic and therapeutic challenge. *Cough*. 2009;5(11):11. http://dx.doi.org/10.1186/1745-9974-5-11. Medline:20015366

Pelucchi C, Grigoryan L, Galeone C, et al, and the ESCMID Sore Throat Guideline Group. Guideline for the management of acute sore throat. *Clin Microbiol Infect*. 2012;18(suppl 1):1–28. http://dx.doi.org/10.1111/j.1469-0691.2012.03766.x. Medline:22432746

Endocrine system

Dr. Launny Faulkner

DISORDERS AND CLINICAL PRESENTATIONS

Adrenal disorders

ADRENAL INSUFFICIENCY

KEYS TO WORKUP

Adrenal insufficiency is usually suspected in patients with the following symptoms:

- fatigue and muscle weakness
- weight loss
- hypotension
- dark tan freckling of the skin
- hypoglycemia
- nausea, vomiting, and diarrhea
- salt craving

There is considerable variation in the approach to the diagnosis of adrenal insufficiency. The goals of testing are to demonstrate inappropriately low levels of cortisol and to determine whether cortisol deficiency is independent of a deficiency in adrenocorticotropic hormone (ACTH). Treatment depends on whether the insufficiency is primary to the adrenal glands (Addison disease), or due to pituitary or hypothalamic dysfunction.

LAB INVESTIGATIONS

See Figure 1.

Start with an early morning (8 a.m.) serum cortisol test. A result of $\geq$ 138 nmol/L (5 µg/dL) makes adrenal insufficiency unlikely.

If the serum cortisol is low, proceed with a serum ACTH level.

- ACTH levels > 66 pmol/L (300 pg/mL) indicate Addison disease.
- ACTH levels < 2.2 pmol/L (10 pg/mL) are consistent with pituitary or hypothalamic failure.

- ACTH levels between 2.2 pmol/L (10 pg/mL) and 66 pmol/L (300 pg/mL) are nondiagnostic.

If ACTH levels are nondiagnostic, proceed to an ACTH (cosyntropin) stimulation test. This consists of baseline (time 0) serum cortisol measurement, and then 250 mg of IM or IV cosyntropin (synthetic ACTH) followed by serum cortisol measurements at 30 and 60 minutes.

- A serum cortisol level > 552 nmol/L (20 µg/dL) at either 30 or 60 minutes is a normal response.
- A serum cortisol level < 138 nmol/L (5 µg/dL) indicates Addison disease.
- A serum cortisol level between 138 nmol/L (5 µg/dL) and 552 nmol/L (20 µg/dL) suggests pituitary failure.

Further testing for adrenal failure may include insulin tolerance testing, adrenal autoantibodies, and 11-deoxycortisol testing. Specialist involvement is recommended if considering these tests.

PEARLS
Once a diagnosis of adrenal insufficiency is made, it is important to seek treatable causes of this disorder. Other tests to consider may include a CT scan or MRI of the adrenal and pituitary glands, a chest X-ray to exclude lung cancer, and tests of the hypothalamic-pituitary axis such as thyroid-stimulating hormone (TSH), prolactin, follicle-stimulating hormone (FSH), and luteinizing hormone (LH).

CUSHING SYNDROME

KEYS TO WORKUP
Cushing syndrome refers to the clinical manifestations of excess cortisol.

Symptoms include:

- weight gain
- stretch marks on the skin of the trunk and arms
- acne
- easy bruising
- fatigue and weakness
- diabetes
- menstrual irregularities
- loss of libido
- depression or anxiety
- hypertension

The causes of excess cortisol include:

- tumours of the pituitary gland, adrenal glands, lung, or pancreas
- exogenous steroids

Cushing disease refers specifically to hypercortisolism caused by an ACTH-secreting pituitary adenoma. Be sure to carefully rule out any exogenous sources of steroids before proceeding with laboratory testing.

LAB INVESTIGATIONS
See Figure 2.

Start with the following tests, which are the most sensitive and specific:

- late-night (11:00) salivary cortisol level
- 24-hour urine free cortisol level

Current guidelines recommend measuring these levels twice.

If either the salivary or urine free cortisol is elevated or equivocal, proceed to a low-dose dexamethasone suppression test. This generally involves administering 1 mg po dexamethasone at 11:00 p.m. and measuring the serum cortisol at 8 a.m. the following morning. A normal response is a serum cortisol level of < 50 nmol/L (1.8 µg/dL).

At least 2 of these 3 tests (salivary cortisol, urine free cortisol, low-dose dexamethasone suppression) must be unequivocally abnormal to make the diagnosis of Cushing syndrome. Once diagnosed, consider further investigations to determine whether cortisol secretion is autonomous (e.g., functioning adrenal tumor) or dependent on ACTH. If dependent, corticotropin-releasing hormone (CRH) stimulation tests can localize the source of ACTH to either the pituitary gland or an ectopic site. However, as these tests are expensive and difficult to interpret, referral to a specialist is recommended.

PEARLS

Cortisol may be elevated in other conditions that are often not readily apparent, such as depression, chronic alcoholism, polycystic ovary syndrome, and eating disorders.

As with Addison disease, imaging of the adrenal and pituitary glands may be indicated.

Diabetes

Symptoms of polyuria and polydipsia may arise from a number of causes, among which are:

- diabetes insipidus (DI): inability to concentrate urine due to decreased quantity or response to antidiuretic hormone (ADH)
- diabetes mellitus: osmotic diuresis secondary to excess urine glucose

DIABETES INSIPIDUS

KEYS TO WORKUP

In the absence of a glucose-induced osmotic diuresis (i.e., uncontrolled diabetes mellitus), there are

3 major causes of polyuria in the outpatient setting (see the breakdown that follows).

Cause	Details
Primary polydipsia	Primary increase in water intake, often secondary to psychiatric illness or medication side effect
Central diabetes insipidus	Deficient secretion of ADH secondary to trauma, hypoxic injury, or idiopathic dysfunction of the pituitary
Nephrogenic diabetes insipidus	Resistance of the renal tubules to ADH; seen in mild form in the elderly and in chronic renal disease; severe resistance usually associated with lithium therapy or hypercalcemia

LAB INVESTIGATIONS
See Figure 3.

Each of the main nondiabetic causes of polyuria is associated with excretion of relatively dilute urine. However, comparison of the plasma sodium concentration and urine osmolality may help distinguish among these disorders.

- A low plasma sodium—less than 137 mmol/L (137 mEq/L)—with a low urine osmolality (e.g., half the plasma osmolality) is indicative of water overload due to primary polydipsia.
- A high-normal plasma sodium—greater than 142 mmol/L (142 mEq/L)—points toward DI, particularly if the urine osmolality is less than the plasma osmolality.
- A normal plasma sodium concentration associated with a urine osmolality of more than 600 mmol/kg (600 mOsmol/kg) excludes a diagnosis of DI.

WATER DEPRIVATION TESTING
Except when the history strongly suggests nephrogenic DI (e.g., long-term lithium use), it is prudent to confirm results via a water deprivation test.

This test involves a supervised period of water restriction and the measurement of:

- urine volume and osmolality every 1 hour
- plasma sodium concentration and osmolality every 2 hours

Overnight fluid restriction with morning measurement is not an acceptable alternative: patients with psychogenic polydipsia may not follow instructions to restrict fluid intake, and those with significant polyuria may become severely volume deplete and hypernatremic.

The supervised test is continued until 1 of the following criteria is met:

- The urine osmolality increases above 600 mmol/kg (600 mOsmol/kg), indicating that both ADH release and effect are intact.
- The urine osmolality is stable on 2 or 3 successive measurements despite a rising plasma osmolality.
- The plasma osmolality exceeds 295–300 mmol/kg (295–300 mOsmol/kg) or the plasma sodium is 145 mmol/L (145 mEq/L) or higher.

In the last 2 settings, desmopressin (synthetic ADH) is administered, and the urine osmolality and volume monitored every 30 minutes over the next 2 hours. A blood sample should be collected immediately prior to the administration of desmopressin so that endogenous ADH levels can be measured if the results are equivocal. Urine ADH testing may be performed if high-sensitivity plasma ADH assays are not available.

INTERPRETATION

Interpret the results of water deprivation testing as follows:

- psychogenic polydipsia: confirmed if urine osmolality reaches a clearly normal value—greater than 500 mmol/kg (500 mOsmol/kg)—with water restriction alone

- central DI: consistent with a submaximal increase in urine osmolality above 300 mmol/kg (300 mOsmol/kg) and confirmed by a rise of more than 100% (complete) or 15% to 50% (partial)
- nephrogenic DI: urine osmolality increases only slightly in response to water deprivation—less than 300 mmol/kg (300 mOsmol/kg)—and desmopressin produces little or no elevation (complete), or a rise not greater than 45% (partial)

If results are borderline or conflicting, send the blood sample—taken before desmopressin was administered—for measurement of endogenous ADH levels.

- Central DI is excluded if an appropriate rise in ADH occurs with the rise in plasma osmolality.
- Nephrogenic DI is excluded if an appropriate rise in urine osmolality occurs as plasma ADH increases.

SOURCES OF ERROR

It is important to monitor for a full 2 hours post desmopressin dose in order to assess response, as any concentrated new urine might be diluted with postmicturitional residual urine (as much as 200 mL to 400 mL).

Patients with partial central DI may be hyperresponsive to the small amounts of ADH induced by water restriction, possibly because of receptor upregulation. Thus, they may be polyuric at normal plasma osmolality but exhibit maximal concentration of urine at higher levels. As desmopressin has little effect in this setting, results may mimic primary polydipsia. To complicate matters further, primary polydipsia may mimic central DI in that chronic overhydration can cause partial suppression of ADH release. As always, clinical history provides important clues, with abrupt onset favouring central DI and gradual onset favouring primary polydipsia.

DIABETES MELLITUS

KEYS TO WORKUP
Type 1 diabetes mellitus is usually diagnosed in childhood or early adulthood. Investigations are triggered by symptoms such as polyuria, polydipsia, fatigue, and weight loss, or are initiated following dramatic presentation with diabetic ketoacidosis (DKA).

Type 2 diabetes mellitus is discovered through routine screening of older, at-risk populations and only rarely through hyperglycemic emergencies. When a patient presents with symptoms that may be associated with diabetes mellitus, the laboratory tests used to make the diagnosis are no different than those used for screening. However, patients showing signs of DKA or hyperosmolar hyperglycemic state (HHS) should be sent to the nearest emergency department for evaluation and appropriate management.

See: routine screening, diabetes, p. 233

LAB INVESTIGATIONS
See Figure 4.[1]

In a patient with symptoms or signs of hyperglycemia, order either:

- HbA_{1c} (preferred initial test for diabetes)
- fasting plasma glucose (when HbA_{1c} is not readily available or is equivocal)

If borderline results are obtained, an oral glucose tolerance test may help distinguish diabetes from "prediabetic" states. In addition, some guidelines state that a random plasma glucose greater than 11.1 mmol/L (200 mg/dL) is diagnostic in a symptomatic patient.

SOURCES OF ERROR

During treatment for diabetes, falsely high values for HbA_{1c} may be obtained in conditions causing decreased red cell turnover and a higher proportion of older red cells (e.g., iron or vitamin B_{12} deficiency). Similarly, rapid red cell turnover leads to a greater proportion of younger red cells and falsely low HbA_{1c} values. Examples include hemolysis, recent treatment of iron or vitamin B_{12} deficiency, and use of erythropoietin.

Some endogenous or exogenous substances may interfere directly with HbA_{1c} testing. For a current list, refer to the website of the National Glycohemoglobin Standardization Program (NGSP).

PEARLS

A HbA_{1c} measurement reflects the average blood glucose concentration over the lifetime of the red blood cells sampled. Thus, it will reflect changes only once a significant population of red cells has turned over. To monitor therapy, therefore, it is recommended that HbA_{1c} testing occur no more frequently than every 3 months.

HbA_{1c} concentrations may be higher in non-Caucasian groups than in Caucasians with similar plasma glucose concentrations. However, these small differences have not been shown to modify the association between HbA_{1c} and clinical outcomes.

Thyroid Disorders

The diagnosis of thyroid disease relies heavily on laboratory tests, as even classical presentations lack specificity. Screening for thyroid disease remains controversial: there is no evidence to indicate that early detection and treatment improves outcomes.

HYPERTHYROIDISM

KEYS TO WORKUP

Patients with primary hyperthyroidism have a suppressed TSH and an elevated free T_4.

Patients with subclinical hyperthyroidism may have a borderline TSH and normal free T_4.

Once the diagnosis of hyperthyroidism has been established, the cause of the hyperthyroidism should be determined. Along with findings on physical exam (e.g., exophthalmos, diffuse goitre), the pattern of abnormal thyroid tests may suggest a specific diagnosis (see Table 3).

Table 3. Causes of hyperthyroidism

Causes of hyperthyroidism can be divided into 2 categories: those that manifest normal or increased uptake on a radioactive iodine scan, and those that manifest decreased or absent uptake.

Process	Specific etiology	Radioactive iodine uptake
Autoimmune disease	Graves disease, Hashimoto thyroiditis	Normal or increased
Autonomous thyroid tissue	Thyroid adenoma, multinodular goitre	
Excess TSH production	Pituitary adenoma	
hCG-related hyperthyroidism	Hyperemesis gravidarum (usually subclinical), trophoblastic disease (hydatidiform mole or choriocarcinoma), paraneoplastic syndrome (rare)	

Continued on p. 34

Continued from p. 33

Process	Specific etiology	Radioactive iodine uptake
Thyroiditis	Subacute granulomatous (de Quervain) thyroiditis, lymphocytic thyroiditis., iatrogenic (radiation, palpation, amiodarone-induced)	Decreased or absent (release of preformed hormone)
Exogenous thyroid hormone	Excessive dosing of thyroxine, natural remedies (e.g., desiccated cow thyroid)	
Ectopic thyroid hormone production	Neoplasm (e.g., struma ovarii) or production from metastatic thyroid cancer	

LAB INVESTIGATIONS

See Figure 5.

The best initial test for the evaluation of hyperthyroidism is a TSH, followed by a free T_4 to confirm the diagnosis.

TESTS FOR PRIMARY HYPERTHYROIDISM

A patient is very unlikely to have primary hyperthyroidism without a suppressed TSH.

However, if the diagnosis is strongly suspected despite a normal TSH:

- It is reasonable to repeat the TSH.
- Measure the free T_4.

Measurement of free T_3 is rarely indicated, and is reserved for situations where hyperthyroidism is suspected and the TSH is suppressed but the free T_4 is normal. This pattern, termed T_3 toxicosis, may occur in Graves disease or multinodular goitre. A radioiodine uptake scan is often important for definitive diagnosis, and is superior to measurement of thyrotropin receptor antibodies.

Most laboratories retain specimens for several days so that follow-up tests can be added without further inconvenience to the patient.

TESTS FOR SUBCLINICAL HYPERTHYROIDISM

The following results together suggest subclinical hyperthyroidism:

- low or low-normal TSH
- normal free T_4 (and T_3)

Most patients have no clinical manifestations or else symptoms that are mild and nonspecific, yet many are ultimately found to have an autonomously functioning adenoma, multinodular goitre, or mild Graves disease.

Patients with a clear cause for subclinical hyperthyroidism are unlikely to normalize spontaneously and are more likely to benefit from treatment, therefore follow-up testing with TSH and free T_4 in 6 to 12 months is recommended.

OTHER TESTS

Patients with hyperthyroidism may have other nonspecific laboratory findings such as:

- low LDL and HDL cholesterol
- normochromic, normocytic anemia
- elevated alkaline phosphatase (due to increased bone turnover)

While these results can support the diagnosis in difficult cases, they are not typically ordered as part of the initial workup.

MONITORING

Pituitary secretion of TSH may be suppressed for prolonged periods following hyperthyroidism. Allow at least 3 months before repeating TSH levels.

If a biochemical measurement of thyroid function is required during this period due to a significant change in clinical status, free T_4 is preferred.

SOURCES OF ERROR

Euthyroid patients with nonthyroidal illness may have low TSH, especially those receiving high-dose steroids or dopamine. Free T_4 is low or low-normal in this population. It is preferable to avoid testing thyroid function in acutely ill patients, but if such results are obtained the patient should be reevaluated in 4 to 8 weeks after the illness has resolved.

Failing to allow enough time for physiologic equilibration is a common source of error in tests of thyroid function. In patients treated for hyperthyroidism or recovering from thyroiditis, TSH concentrations may remain low for several months after normalization of T_4 and T_3.

There is considerable debate over what constitutes the "true" normal range for TSH, especially in older adults. In otherwise healthy elderly patients, an altered set point of the hypothalamic-pituitary-thyroid axis may cause TSH concentrations outside the normal range.

PEARLS

Patients with thyrotoxicosis (the clinical syndrome caused by hyperthyroidism) usually have a TSH value < 0.1 mIU/L. However, in the setting of a TSH-producing pituitary adenoma, hyperthyroidism is secondary to an excess of TSH. The combination of elevated TSH and free T_4 may also be seen in partial resistance to thyroid hormone, whereby the feedback of T_4 and T_3 to the pituitary is disrupted.

Rarely, patients presenting with symptoms of hypothyroidism have a low TSH and low or low-normal free T_4, indicating a central cause (pituitary or hypothalamus) of thyroid dysfunction.

HYPOTHYROIDISM

KEYS TO WORKUP

Primary hypothyroidism is characterized by a high TSH concentration and a low free T_4 concentration.

Subclinical hypothyroidism is defined as a normal free T_4 concentration in the presence of an elevated TSH.

Central hypothyroidism is much less common, and is characterized by a low T_4 concentration with a TSH that is not appropriately elevated (may be low, normal, or only mildly elevated). In this setting, differentiation must be made between pituitary (secondary hypothyroidism) and hypothalamic (tertiary hypothyroidism) disorders. Signs and symptoms of additional hormone disturbances support a diagnosis of central hypothyroidism.

See Table 4 for causes of hypothyroidism.

Table 4. Causes of hypothyroidism

Process	Specific etiology
Autoimmune disease	Chronic autoimmune thyroiditis (subacute granulomatous, lymphocytic, postpartum)
Iatrogenic	Thyroidectomy, radioactive iodine therapy or external radiation
Infiltrative disease	Fibrous thyroiditis, hemochromatosis, sarcoidosis
Drugs	Withdrawal of high dose thyroxine
	Thionamides, lithium, amiodarone, perchlorate, immunologics
Congenital	Thyroid agenesis, dysgenesis, or defects in hormone synthesis
	Generalized thyroid hormone resistance
Central hypothyroidism	TSH or TRH deficiency secondary to pituitary or hypothalamic insult (injury, infarct, infection, neoplasm)

LAB INVESTIGATIONS

See Figure 5.

TSH is the single best initial test for the investigation of patients with symptoms or signs of hypothyroidism.

- If the TSH is elevated, order a repeat TSH to rule out transient elevation from another cause, along with a free T_4 to confirm the diagnosis.
- If the TSH remains elevated but the T_4 is normal, this may indicate subclinical hypothyroidism. Decisions about T_4 replacement must be made on a case-by-case basis.
- If the patient has convincing symptoms of hypothyroidism despite an initially normal TSH, order a repeat TSH and free T_4 to assess for central hypothyroidism. Low free T_3 is seen in severe hypothyroidism, but measurement of free T_3 is generally not indicated in the investigation of hypothyroidism.

NOT RECOMMENDED

Testing for anti–thyroid peroxidase antibodies (anti-TPO) is sometimes done to confirm a suspected autoimmune cause of hypothyroidism. However, since the presence of anti-TPO antibodies does not affect disease management, this test has little clinical utility.

ABOUT MONITORING

TSH values change very slowly. Retest TSH levels no sooner than 8 to 12 weeks following a change in thyroxine replacement or the patient's clinical status. Once target values are within the normal euthyroid range, and once the TSH has stabilized, an annual level is sufficient for monitoring therapy.

TSH is only a useful measure of thyroid disease when the hypothalamic-pituitary-thyroid axis is intact. When central disease is suspected, free T_4 measurement is preferred to assess adequacy of thyroid replacement therapy.

SOURCES OF ERROR

As with many immunoassays, the presence of certain antibodies in the patient's serum may interfere with measurement. These include:

- autoantibodies to TSH
- heterophile antibodies against mouse antibodies (common in patients previously treated with immunologics)
- rheumatoid factor

False-positive results are most common, with a spuriously elevated TSH but normal free T_4.

If you suspect interference by an antibody, inform the lab so it can take steps to circumvent or eliminate this problem. As always, consultation with a lab director is recommended when a test result conflicts with the clinical presentation.

See also: hyperthyroidism, sources of error, p. 36

PEARLS

Euthyroid patients with nonthyroidal illness may have transient elevations in TSH concentrations. In patients with a recent illness, TSH and free T_4 should be measured 4 to 6 weeks after recovery.

Rare causes of elevated TSH include resistance to thyroid hormone and TSH-producing pituitary adenomas. In both cases the free T_4 will also be elevated, producing variable symptoms of hyperthyroidism.

There is considerable debate over what constitutes the "true" normal range for TSH, especially in older adults. In otherwise healthy elderly patients, an altered set point of the hypothalamic-pituitary-thyroid axis may cause TSH concentrations outside the normal range.

REFERENCES

1 Ekoé JM, Punthakee Z, Ransom T, Prebtani APH, Goldenberg R; Canadian Diabetes Association Clinical Practice Guidelines Expert Committee. Screening for type 1 and type 2 diabetes. *Can J Diabetes* 2013;37(suppl 1):S12–15. http://dx.doi.org/10.1016/j.jcjd.2013.01.012

FURTHER READING

British Columbia Ministry of Health Services, Guidelines and Protocols Advisory Committee. Thyroid function tests: diagnoses and monitoring of thyroid disorders in adults. www.bcguidelines.ca/pdf/thyroid.pdf. January 1, 2010.

Toward Optimized Practice Program. Clinical practice guideline: investigation and management of primary thyroid dysfunction. October 2005. www.topalbertadoctors.org/download/350/thyroid_guideline.pdf. Updated 2008.

Figure 1. Diagnostic algorithm for adrenal insufficiency

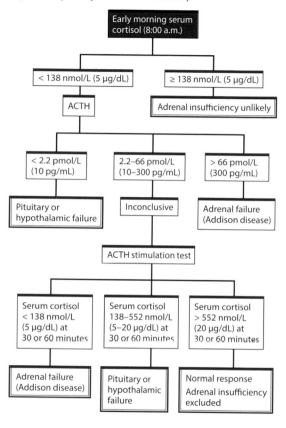

Figure 2. Diagnostic algorithm for Cushing syndrome

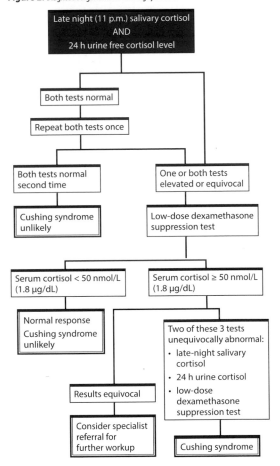

Figure 3. Diagnostic algorithm for polyuria and polydipsia

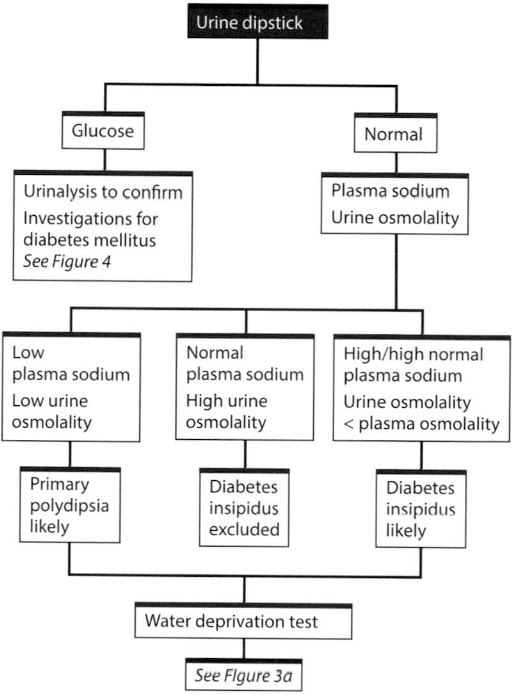

Figure 3a

(Figure 3 continued)

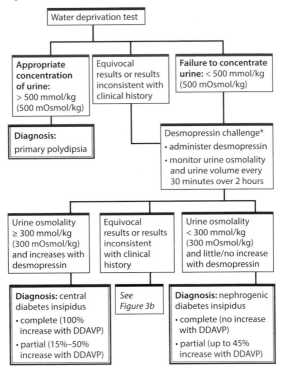

*Desmopressin should not be given before the urine osmolality has stabilized or the plasma osmolality has reached 295 mmol/kg (295 mOsmol/kg), otherwise the accuracy of the desmopressin challenge may be affected.

Figure 3b

(Figure 3a continued)

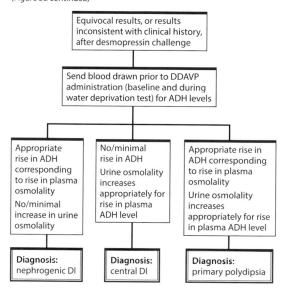

Figure 4. Diagnostic algorithm for diabetes mellitus

This figure presents the guidelines of the Canadian Diabetes Association, in SI units. Other guidelines may apply in other jurisdictions.

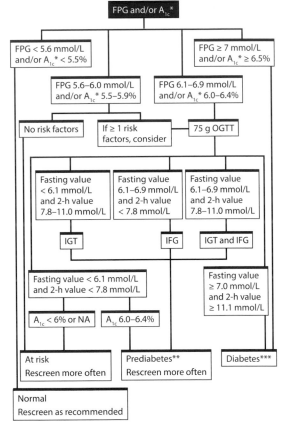

*HbA$_{1c}$ is preferred. If both fasting plasma glucose (FPG) and glycated hemoglobin (A$_{1c}$) are available but discordant, use the HbA$_{1c}$.

**Prediabetes = impaired fasting glucose (IFG), impaired glucose tolerance (IGT), or A$_{1c}$ 6.0% to 6.4%

***In the absence of symptomatic hyperglycemia, if a single laboratory test is in the diabetes range, a repeat confirmatory test (FPG, A$_{1c}$, 2hPG in a 75 g OGTT) must be done on another day. It is preferable that the same test be repeated (in a timely fashion) for confirmation. If results of 2 different tests are available and both are above the diagnostic cutpoints, the diagnosis of diabetes is confirmed.

Figure 5. Diagnostic algorithm for disorders of thyroid function

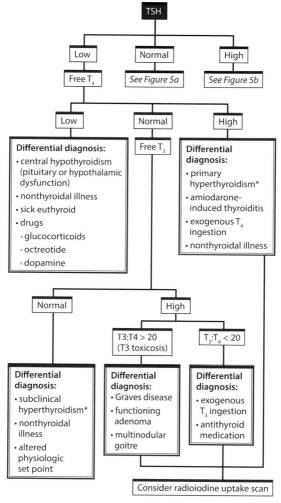

*For etiologies of hyperthyroidism, see Table 3.

Figure 5a

(Figure 5 continued)

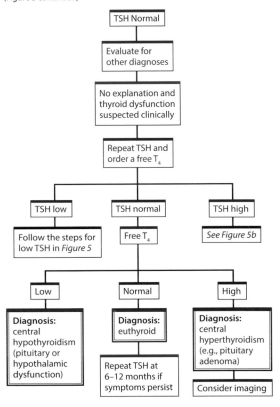

Figure 5b

(Figure 5a continued)

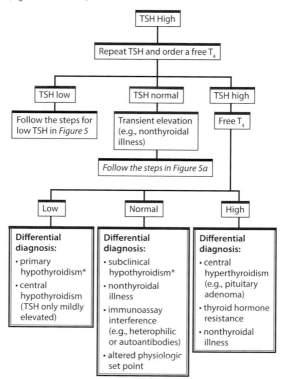

*For etiologies of hypothyroidism, see Table 4.

Figure 5c. Therapeutic monitoring in disorders of thyroid function

(Figure 5b continued)

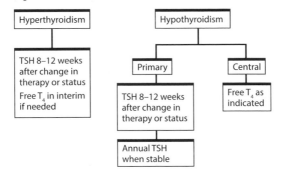

Fatigue

Dr. Christopher Naugler

ABBREVIATIONS

ALP	alkaline phosphatase	GGT	γ-glutamyltransferase
ALT	alanine aminotransferase	HbA$_{1c}$	glycated hemoglobin
ANA	antinuclear antibody	MCHC	mean corpuscular hemoglobin concentration
AST	aspartate aminotransferase		
CBC	complete blood count	MCV	mean corpuscular volume
CKMB	creatine kinase MB	NT-pro BNP	N-terminal prohormone of brain natriuretic peptide
COPD	chronic obstructive pulmonary disease		
		PT/INR	prothrombin time or international normalized ratio
CRP	C-reactive protein		
eGFR	estimated glomerular filtration rate	RF	rheumatoid factor
		T$_3$	triiodothyronine
ESR	erythrocyte sedimentation rate	T$_4$	thyroxine
FSH	follicle-stimulating hormone	TSH	thyroid-stimulating hormone (thyrotropin)
FIT	fecal immunochemical test		
gFOBT	guaiac fecal occult blood test		

OVERALL APPROACH

Common causes of fatigue

Fatigue is a very common presenting complaint, especially in the context of primary care. It has a broad differential diagnosis (see Table 5). The starting point is a careful and thorough history and physical exam.

Certain signs, symptoms, and factors deserve particular attention, including:

- psychological and social problems
- pain and other musculoskeletal problems
- respiratory symptoms, including reactive airways disease and chronic obstructive pulmonary disease (COPD)
- bladder and bowel problems
- cardiovascular disease

Table 5. Common causes of fatigue

Category	Specific etiologies
Cardiovascular	Congestive heart failure
	Angina pectoris
Digestive	Diarrhea
	Constipation
	Celiac disease
	Liver disease
Endocrine	Hyper-/hypothyroidism
	Hyperparathyroidism
	Diabetes mellitus
	Obesity
	Menopause
	Bone disease
Musculoskeletal	Arthritis
	Nerve entrapment
	Polymyalgia rheumatica
Neurologic	Headache
	Postconcussion syndrome
Psychological	Depression
	Anxiety
	Social problems

Continued on p. 53

Continued from p. 52

Category	Specific etiologies
Respiratory	Asthma
	COPD
	Chronic cough
	Hypoxia
Systemic	Anemia
	Renal failure
	Medication side effect
	Allergy
	Chronic pain syndrome
	Chronic fatigue syndrome
	Malignancy
	Chronic itch
	Hepatitis

Role of laboratory testing

Laboratory tests have a low yield for identifying causes of fatigue.

For patients presenting with fatigue, you can generally begin with a 1-month period of observation before ordering tests, unless symptoms point to a specific diagnosis or you find warning signs such as weight loss, fever, or pain.

DISORDERS AND CLINICAL PRESENTATIONS

ANEMIA AND FATIGUE

KEYS TO WORKUP

If clinical evidence and observation point to anemia, begin with a CBC and base further investigations on the CBC results.

If the patient is anemic, look at the mean corpuscular volume (MCV) and mean corpuscular hemoglobin concentration (MCHC). This will separate the anemia into:

- normocytic: common causes include acute blood loss, chronic disease
- microcytic: common causes include iron deficiency, sideroblastic anemia, and possibly chronic disease
- macrocytic: common causes include myelodysplastic syndromes, vitamin B_{12} deficiency, alcoholism, and drug effects

Note that folate deficiency can cause macrocytic anemia, but it is very rare in Canada since the universal supplementation of flour began several decades ago. It is generally unnecessary to test for folate deficiency.

LAB INVESTIGATIONS

CBC
Remember that hemoglobin levels have age and sex specific normal ranges.

FERRITIN
A microcytic hypochromic anemia with concomitant low ferritin is characteristic of iron deficiency anemia. Remember, however, that ferritin may be an acute phase reactant and may therefore be elevated or in the normal range if there is a coexistent inflammatory disorder.

PEARLS
Iron deficiency anemia in an older individual should always raise the suspicion of colonic carcinoma. These patients warrant colonoscopy. A fecal immunochemical test (FIT) is sometimes used as an initial screen in these patients, depending on local availability of colonoscopy. Note that FIT is superior to the traditional guaiac fecal occult blood test (gFOBT)—gFOBT is being phased out.

See also: anemia, p. 134

CARDIOVASCULAR SYMPTOMS AND FATIGUE

KEYS TO WORKUP

Clinical presentation should guide decisions about laboratory testing.

LAB INVESTIGATIONS

HIGH SENSITIVITY TROPONIN

In cases of suspected acute coronary syndrome, high sensitivity troponin is the preferred test to creatine kinase MB (CKMB).

Commonly used reference ranges for high sensitivity troponin T are:

- negative: ≤ 14 ng/L (0.14 ng/mL)
- borderline elevation: 15–109 ng/L (0.15– 1.09 ng/mL)
- clear elevation: ≥ 110 ng/L (1.10 ng/mL)

NT-PRO BNP

This test can support a diagnosis of congestive heart failure in equivocal cases.

Heart failure is unlikely if:

- NT-pro BNP is < 300 ng/L (300 pg/mL)

Heart failure is likely if:

- NT-pro BNP is > 450 ng/L (450 pg/mL) for patients < 50 years of age
- NT-pro BNP is > 900 ng/L (900 pg/mL) for patients 50–75 years of age
- NT-pro BNP is > 1800 ng/L (1800 pg/mL) for patients > 75 years of age

PEARLS

The reference range for BNP differs from NT-pro BNP: always refer to your local laboratory reference ranges for any blood test.

Troponin I, troponin T, and high sensitivity troponin T have different reference ranges. The interpretation of troponin levels is the focus of much current research.

CHRONIC FATIGUE SYNDROME

Chronic fatigue syndrome is diagnosed clinically. There are no diagnostic laboratory findings.

Note that diagnosis of this entity can be difficult and controversial.

CLIMACTERIC (MENOPAUSAL) SYMPTOMS AND FATIGUE

KEYS TO WORKUP

Laboratory testing is generally unnecessary: the absence of menstruation confirms the diagnosis for most patients.

LAB INVESTIGATIONS

If there is clinical confusion with a possible diagnosis of hypothyroidism, then the situation may warrant the following panel of tests:

- estradiol (E_2)
- follicle-stimulating hormone (FSH)
- thyroid-stimulating hormone (TSH)

Increased FSH and decreased estradiol levels are characteristic of menopause.

FATIGUE WITHOUT LOCALIZING OR ACCOMPANYING SYMPTOMS

KEYS TO WORKUP

If clinical evidence and observation do not point to a diagnosis, a panel of tests can help narrow the diagnosis.

Abnormalities in any of the tests may point to a specific etiology and trigger further investigations. In the absence of any positive findings, consider other causes such as psychological and social problems.

LAB INVESTIGATIONS

If needed, order the tests in the breakdown that follows as a panel.

Tests	Diagnostic value
ALP	Liver disease
ALT	
AST	
Direct and indirect bilirubin	
GGT	
PT/INR	
CBC	Anemia
CRP	Autoimmune disease
	Malignancy
Glucose or Hb$_{A1c}$	Diabetes
Calcium	Bone disease
	Malignancy
	Hyperparathyroidism
Creatinine/eGFR	Renal failure
TSH	Hyper-/hypothyroidism

PEARLS

Best-practice recommendations are largely lacking for the investigation of these patients.

An erythrocyte sedimentation rate (ESR) does not add useful additional information to the CRP result for most patients.

Vitamin B$_{12}$ is not a useful initial screening test unless the patient has known intestinal malabsorption or macrocytic anemia.

HYPOTHYROIDISM AND FATIGUE

KEYS TO WORKUP

If clinical evidence and observation point to hypothyroidism, begin with a TSH level.

LAB INVESTIGATIONS

TSH

This is the single best initial test for the investigation of patients with symptoms or signs of hypothyroidism.

REPEAT TSH WITH FREE T$_4$

This is a follow-up test:

- if initial TSH is elevated
- if fatigue persists

If you suspect fatigue symptoms are due to subclinical hypothyroidism (common in older individuals), a repeat TSH and free T$_4$ in 6 months is often useful in clarifying the diagnosis.

NOT RECOMMENDED

T$_3$ and reverse T$_3$ are not generally useful in the evaluation of thyroid function in the community setting.

See: hypothyroidism, p. 37

MUSCULOSKELETAL DISORDERS AND FATIGUE

KEYS TO TESTING

Findings from history and physical examination should guide decisions about laboratory tests.

Insomnia secondary to arthritic pain may not require testing: history and clinical presentation are often sufficient for these patients.

LAB INVESTIGATIONS

Consider the following tests in cases of inflammatory arthritis or new arthritis associated with other systemic symptoms:

- antinuclear antibody (ANA)
  - Positive ANA results may indicate diseases such as systemic lupus erythematosus, systemic sclerosis, other autoimmune diseases, and malignancies.

- ° A positive ANA test, however, is not specific and may be positive in up to 5% of normal individuals.

- CBC
- CRP
  - ° This is neither a sensitive nor specific marker of inflammation. However, levels above 10 mg/L (1.0 mg/dL) are generally consistent with active inflammation or malignancy.

- HLA-B27
- rheumatoid factor (RF)
  - ° An elevated RF is present in most individuals with rheumatoid arthritis, but may also be found in up to 20% of healthy older individuals.

PEARLS
HLA-B27 is strongly associated with ankylosing spondylitis; however, most individuals with the HLA-B27 allele will not suffer from this disorder.

PSYCHOLOGICAL DISORDERS AND FATIGUE
There are no diagnostic laboratory findings.
See: neuropsychiatry, p. 211

RESPIRATORY SYMPTOMS AND FATIGUE
KEYS TO WORKUP
There are no diagnostic laboratory findings for respiratory symptoms.

PEARLS
Diagnosis of reactive airways disease and COPD is based on:

- history
- physical exam
- abnormalities on pulmonary function testing and (possibly) related X-ray findings

Immunoglobulin testing for specific allergens has low sensitivity and specificity, and is generally unnecessary.

SORE THROAT AND FATIGUE

KEYS TO WORKUP

Fatigue accompanied by a sore throat raises the possibility of infectious mononucleosis. Less commonly, this presentation signals immunodeficiency or leukemia, or other malignancy. A careful history and a thorough physical examination are key to sorting out these diagnoses.

LAB INVESTIGATIONS

Order the following tests as a panel:

- CBC
- heterophile antibody test (mono test): note that this test may be negative during the initial infection period (first 2 weeks) of infectious mononucleosis
- peripheral blood smear: this test can be very useful in supporting a diagnosis of infectious mononucleosis and ruling out more serious causes

FURTHER READING

Hamilton W, Watson J, Round A. Investigating fatigue in primary care. *BMJ*. 2010;341:c4259. http://dx.doi.org/10.1136/bmj.c4259. Medline:20736254

Nijrolder I, van der Windt D, de Vries H, et al. Diagnoses during follow-up of patients presenting with fatigue in primary care. *CMAJ*. 2009;181(10):683–687. http://dx.doi.org/10.1503/cmaj.090647. Medline:19858240

Adlin V. Subclinical hypothyroidism: deciding when to treat. *Am Fam Physician*. 1998;57(4):776–780. Medline:9491000

Gastrointestinal and hepatic system

Dr. Ethan Flynn

ABBREVIATIONS

ABG	arterial blood gas	eGFR	estimated glomerular filtration rate
AFP	α_1-fetoprotein		
ALP	alkaline phosphatase	EIA	enzyme immunoassay
ALT	alanine aminotransferase	ELISA	enzyme-linked immunosorbent assay
AMA	antimitochondrial antibodies		
ANA	antinuclear antibody	EMA	antiendomysial antibody
ALKM-1	anti–liver kidney microsomal antibody type 1	ERCP	endoscopic retrograde cholangiopancreatography
aPTT	activated partial thromboplastin time	ESR	erythrocyte sedimentation rate
		GERD	gastroesophageal reflux disease
ASMA	anti–smooth muscle antibody	gFOBT	guaiac fecal occult blood test
AST	aspartate aminotransferase	FIT	fecal immunochemical test
BUN	blood urea nitrogen (serum urea nitrogen)	GGT	γ-glutamyltransferase
		GI	gastrointestinal
CA 125	cancer antigen 125	HAV	hepatitis A virus
CA 19-9	cancer antigen 19-9	Hb	hemoglobin
CBC	complete blood count	HBV	hepatitis B virus
CRP	C-reactive protein	HBcAb	hepatitis B core antibody
CT	computed tomography	HBeAb	hepatitis B e antibody
DIC	disseminated intravascular coagulation	HBsAb	hepatitis B surface antibody
		HBsAg	hepatitis B surface antigen
DKA	diabetic ketoacidosis	hCG	human chorionic gonadotropin
EGD	esophagogastroduodenoscopy	Hct	hematocrit

HCV	hepatitis C virus	PBC	primary biliary cirrhosis
HEV	hepatitis E virus	PCR	polymerase chain reaction
HIV	human immunodeficiency virus	PSC	primary sclerosing cholangitis
IBD	inflammatory bowel disease	PT/INR	prothrombin time or international normalized ratio
IFA	immunofluorescent assay		
IgA	immunoglobulin A	RAST	radioallergosorbent test
IgG	immunoglobulin G	RBC	red blood cell
IgM	immunoglobulin M	RDW	red blood cell distribution width
IV	intravenous	SAAG	serum-ascites albumin gradient
KUB	kidneys, ureter, bladder X-ray	T_3	triiodothyronine
LDH	lactate dehydrogenase	T_4	thyroxine
MCV	mean corpuscular volume	TIBC	total iron binding capacity
MRI	magnetic resonance imaging	TSH	thyroid-stimulating hormone (thyrotropin)
O+P	ova and parasites		
p-ANCA	perinuclear antineutrophil cytoplasmic antibody	tTG	tissue transglutaminase
		WBC	white blood cell

OVERALL APPROACH

Key steps in diagnosis

A well-formulated differential diagnosis is key to identifying gastrointestinal (GI) disorders and comes first from:

- a detailed clinical history
- a thorough physical exam of the abdomen and the body as a whole (e.g., evaluate conjunctivae or skin for jaundice, examine anorectal area for fissures of Crohn disease)

These steps lead to a working clinical differential diagnosis, which determines diagnostic imaging and laboratory testing to rule in or out possible causes and diseases.[1]

Urgent versus nonurgent symptoms

It is also helpful to distinguish symptoms potentially related to gastrointestinal disease that warrant immediate medical care, and symptoms that may not warrant such urgent care but require medical evaluation (see Table 6).

Table 6. Urgent and nonurgent symptoms related to GI disorders

Urgent: require immediate care	Nonurgent: require evaluation
Abdominal pain, extreme	Heartburn (acid reflux)*
GI symptoms with high fever	GI symptoms with persistent low-grade fever
Diarrhea, extreme and lasting more than 1 day	Bloated feeling after eating very little*
Rectal bleeding, moderate to severe	Nausea*
GI symptoms with chest, neck, shoulder, or jaw pain	Chronic diarrhea, watery
Vomiting blood or "coffee ground" material	Belching*
Absent bowel sounds	Abdominal pain, nonextreme
GI symptoms with disorientation or confusion	Acute diarrhea, watery
Guarding, rigidity, or rebound tenderness	Malodorous stools
GI symptoms with significantly decreased or rapid heart rate	Upset stomach*
	Frequent bowel movements
	Colicky postprandial abdominal pain
	Clay-coloured (acholic) stools
	Blood in stool, blood in diarrhea
	Weight loss, unexplained
	Jaundice
	Vomiting
	Chronic diarrhea, bloody
	Flatulence*
	Abdominal cramps
	Inability to have bowel movement, no abdominal pain*
	Indigestion*
	Ascites
	Constipation*

*laboratory workup of little or no utility

Role of laboratory testing

Laboratory testing:

- can help establish the diagnosis and also gauge the clinical severity of the disorder (e.g., severity of GI hemorrhage, end-organ dysfunction due to shock) in conjunction with other diagnostic procedures (e.g., radiology or invasive procedures, as indicated)
- is more efficacious in acute GI disturbances (particularly in the emergency or urgent-care setting)
- is also useful in the outpatient setting in chronic or indolent GI conditions (the latter often in conjunction with endoscopy and endoscopic biopsy with histopathologic evaluation)

DISORDERS AND CLINICAL PRESENTATIONS

ABDOMINAL DISTENSION

KEYS TO WORKUP

The clinical differential diagnosis for abdominal distension is broad and includes:

- ascites (*see: ascites, p. 69*)
- organomegaly (liver, spleen)
- bowel obstruction
- parasitic infestations
- intestinal dysmotility disorder
- celiac disease
- bloating due to high-fibre diet or lactose intolerance
- occult underlying neoplasm (such as ovarian or colon cancer)

Findings from clinical history and physical examination, in conjunction with radiologic studies, should guide laboratory testing.

Note that:

- There may be no need for laboratory testing in patients who are well clinically, and whose abdominal distention has a clear cause on clinical history and physical examination.
- Lab tests are typically performed in patients with abdominal distension whose cause is not readily apparent from clinical evaluation.

LAB INVESTIGATIONS

CBC

This can rule out eosinophilia, which may arise from eosinophilic gastroenteritis or parasitic infestations; it is also indicated if abdominal distension is accompanied by abdominal pain, presenting as "acute abdomen" with distension, since an elevated WBC count is often seen with inflammation or infection.

ALBUMIN

Patients with hypoalbuminemia typically have albumin levels below 25 g/L (2.5 g/dL).

Hypoalbuminemia results in a loss of oncotic pressure and subsequent shift of fluids out of the vasculature and into the peritoneal cavity.

β-hCG

Always order this test for females of childbearing age with abdominal distension. Unsuspected pregnancy is a common cause of abdominal distension in reproductive-age women.

CELIAC DISEASE SEROLOGIES

Order the following tests if celiac disease is suspected:

- IgA tTG antibody (tTG)
- IgA antiendomysial antibody (EMA)
- total IgA level

This test excludes IgA-deficient patients.

IgA-deficient patients may have false-negative results in testing for IgA tTG antibodies (and any other celiac serology evaluating the IgA antibody fraction). These patients require evaluation of the IgG tTG antibody fraction. Note that children younger than 3 with celiac disease may not show elevated tTG or EMA levels.[2]

The American Gastroenterological Association (as opposed to the Canadian Celiac Association) recommends testing for total IgA level only in patients with negative serology in whom celiac disease is strongly suspected clinically. Since IgA deficiency occurs in only 3% or less of patients with celiac disease, this strategy might save money.[3]

FURTHER TESTS FOR CELIAC DISEASE
All patients with strong clinical indications of celiac disease warrant intestinal biopsy regardless of their serology results, because false-negative serological tests can occur. Obtain biopsy specimens before patients start a gluten-free diet, to avoid false-negative biopsy results.

Serology and duodenal mucosal biopsy together are the best way to establish a diagnosis of celiac disease. Use both, not one without the other, to make a definitive diagnosis.

If the diagnosis remains unclear after serology and duodenal mucosal biopsy, consider testing for HLA-DQ2 (95% of celiac patients) and HLA-DQ8 (5% of celiac patients). Patients without DQA1 or DQB1 alleles are virtually guaranteed **not** to have celiac disease.

IgA or IgG antigliadin antibody tests are no longer recommended as screening tests for celiac disease because of their very poor positive and negative predictive values.[4]

TUMOUR MARKERS
Use these tests if intra-abdominal carcinoma is suspected:

- α_1-fetoprotein (AFP)
- cancer antigen 125 (CA 125)
- cancer antigen 19-9 (CA 19-9)

FIT AND gFOBT
The fecal immunochemical test (FIT) and guaiac fecal occult blood test (gFOBT) are used to screen for colonic carcinoma. Positive findings should prompt colonoscopy. Note that FIT is superior to gFOBT (gFOBT is being phased out).

Note that:

- False positives and negatives may occur with either test, but particularly with gFOBT.
- gFOBT has a faster turnaround time than FIT, but has the following limitations:
  - gFOBT has false-negative results with vitamin C supplements, and false-positive results with certain foods.
  - In contrast to FIT, which is an automated test, gFOBT is a visual read: technologists can face challenges in distinguishing positive and negative results.
- FIT is more sensitive (and superior) to gFOBT: it detects as little as 0.3 mL of daily blood loss (as opposed to 10 mL for gFOBT).
- A single gFOBT has a relatively low sensitivity (up to 30%), but 3 consecutive gFOBTs, or

2 consecutive FITs, have a sensitivity of 80%; the specificity is 98% to 99%.

PEARLS

Distension is typically caused by the **5 Fs**: fat, flatus, fluid, fetus, frightful big mass.

ABDOMINAL PAIN, COLICKY POSTPRANDIAL

KEYS TO WORKUP

Dull, constant pain occurring within 1 hour of a meal is most likely due to:

- gallstone(s) impacting the cystic duct of the gallbladder

This causes pain with gallbladder contraction (cholecystitis). Frequently, patients also experience referred pain to the shoulder blade or, when peritoneal inflammation is present, to the right upper quadrant.

Other possible causes of abdominal pain with referred pain include:

- appendicitis
- pancreatitis
- gastroenteritis
- peptic ulcer disease
- bile duct and pancreatic disorders (benign and malignant tumors, strictures)

Note that gastroesophageal reflux disease (GERD) may cause postprandial pain.

Laboratory testing is helpful in determining degree of inflammation and probability of infection (e.g., WBC count in CBC), and may help localize the site of disease (e.g., lipase elevation in ampulla stricture).

LAB INVESTIGATIONS

INITIAL TESTS

Use the following as a panel of initial tests:

- CBC
- amylase
- lipase
- liver function tests: ALP, ALT, GGT, direct and indirect bilirubin

INTERPRETATION

Common bile duct obstruction initially causes an increase in liver-associated enzymes (AST, ALT, GGT) followed a few hours later by increasing bilirubin. AST and ALT begin to fall after a few days with a concomitant steady increase in bilirubin and ALP.

Increase in amylase and lipase implies a blockage or stricture at the ampulla or pancreatic duct.

Elevated WBC count, particularly neutrophilia, suggests ascending cholangitis or other cause of significant inflammation and/or infection.

BLOOD CULTURE

Use this as a follow-up test if WBC (and particularly neutrophil count) is elevated. Blood cultures are positive in one-third to one-half of patients with ascending cholangitis.[5]

ACHOLIC STOOLS

See: jaundice, p. 86

ASCITES

KEYS TO WORKUP

Ascites may be due to:

- primary hepatic causes: alcoholic hepatitis, acute liver failure, biliary disease, Budd-Chiari

syndrome, cirrhosis, hepatocellular adenoma, hepatorenal syndrome, portal hypertension, primary biliary cirrhosis, viral hepatitis
- losses of serum protein: nephrotic syndrome, protein losing enteropathies, severe protein calorie malnutrition (kwashiorkor)
- carcinomatosis (especially ovarian cancer in females)

Lab testing of peripheral blood and peritoneal fluid is valuable in characterizing the properties (and potentially etiology) of ascites (peritoneal effusion).

LAB INVESTIGATIONS

BLOOD CHEMISTRY

Liver function tests should be performed in all cases of new presentation of ascites:

- ALP
- ALT
- AST
- GGT
- PT/INR

Note that elevated PT/INR in a patient not on a PT-elevating drug (e.g., Coumadin/warfarin) may point toward clotting factor deficiency in patients with end-stage liver disease (since almost all clotting factors are made in the liver).

The following tests are useful in further clarifying the etiology or clinical status of patients with ascites:

- BUN and creatinine/eGFR: for coexistent kidney dysfunction or dehydration
- CBC: for associated inflammation or infection
- electrolytes: for metabolic abnormalities related to ascites
- LDH (in conjunction with ascites fluid LDH)
- serum albumin and total protein

Note that hypoalbuminemia results in a loss of oncotic pressure and subsequent shift of fluids out of the vasculature and into the peritoneal cavity. Patients with hypoalbuminemia typically have albumin levels below 25 g/L (2.5 g/dL).

TUMOUR MARKERS

Tumour markers are more helpful in monitoring patients with known malignancy, but may be useful as an adjunct in evaluating patients with suspected malignant effusion (ascites). Use these as clinically indicated:

- AFP
- CA 19-9
- CA 125

VIRAL HEPATITIS PANEL

Use the following tests if findings suggest viral hepatitis:

- hepatitis B core antibody (anti-HBcAb, IgG)
- hepatitis B surface antigen (HBsAg)
- hepatitis B surface antibody (anti-HBsAb)
- hepatitis C antibody (anti-HCV)
- HIV (in at-risk populations, to rule out HIV cholangiopathy)

Examples of clinical indications for testing include:

- patients with history predisposing to viral hepatitis
  - IV drug abuse
  - history of travel to hepatitis-endemic areas
  - at-risk sexual behaviour
- patients with significantly elevated liver-associated enzymes and ascites
- patients with jaundice and ascites

NOT INDICATED

See the breakdown that follows.

Test	Notes
Hepatitis A virus (HAV)	Not indicated for ascites, since viral hepatitis–associated ascites typically occurs after longstanding chronic viral hepatitis with resultant cirrhosis and liver failure, which is not a consequence of the self-limited infection from HAV
Anti-HBeAb and HBeAg	Not recommended in the initial laboratory workup of suspected viral hepatitis (they are used to assess HBV disease severity and for treatment eligibility and/or monitoring)
Hepatitis E virus (HEV)	HEV is not endemic to Canada or the US
	Test for HEV (serology for anti-HEV antibodies) only if the patient has travelled to, or has had contact with persons from, countries where HEV is endemic[6]

Note that:

- Viral hepatitis testing is generally not indicated in patients presenting with clinically obvious carcinomatosis and ascites.
- Anti-HBc IgM is frequently not included in viral hepatitis testing protocols because there is usually no window between disappearance of HBsAg and serologic evidence of resolved infection.

PERITONEAL FLUID

Peritoneal fluid (ascites) lab testing is particularly valuable in evaluating the etiology of ascites (e.g., increased fluid protein in exudative effusion; cancer cells found in cytologic evaluation of fluid) and whether the fluid is infected.

Order the following as a panel:

- cell count and differential: > 250 neutrophils/mm^3 (250/μL) is strongly suggestive of bacterial peritonitis; RBC count > 100 000/mm^3 (100 000/μL) is strongly suggestive of abdominal trauma

- albumin
- total protein
- Gram stain and culture: this may require evaluation of repeat samples if bacterial peritonitis is clinically suspected, to improve sensitivity
- cytology: this rules out malignant effusion (58% to 75% sensitivity); it may require evaluation of repeat samples, if ascites are clinically suspected
- colour and quality (amber, bloody, cloudy, purulent)
- glucose: this may be decreased in infections or other causes of exudative pleural effusions (e.g., malignancy)
- specific gravity: this may be elevated in exudative pleural effusions
- LDH: > 200 U/L in peritoneal fluid implies exudative effusion; in ascites, the ascites fluid LDH:serum LDH ratio is about 0.4 in uncomplicated cirrhosis and typically greater than 1.0 in tumour, infection, or bowel perforation
- amylase: this may be increased in pancreatitis or bowel perforation

PEARLS

The best test (97% accurate) for evaluating portal-hypertensive from nonportal-hypertensive ascites is the serum-ascites albumin gradient (SAAG)[7]:

- SAAG ≥ 1.1: portal-hypertensive-associated
- SAAG < 1.1: nonportal-hypertensive-associated

Laboratory evaluation of ascites is typically done in parallel with radiologic evaluation (KUB studies; abdominal CT and/or ultrasound and/or MRI).

BLOODY DIARRHEA OR STOOL, ACUTE

KEYS TO WORKUP

In cases of mucoid, bloody diarrhea with abrupt onset, laboratory tests help:

- distinguish the etiology of colitis (primarily by establishing an infectious etiology, or supporting allergic or IBD-associated etiologies in the setting of negative stool culture or microscopy)
- identify causative species and antibiotic sensitivities of bacterial colitis

LAB INVESTIGATIONS

TESTS FOR INITIAL WORKUP

See the breakdown that follows.

Test	Notes
CBC	An elevated WBC is often seen with enterohemorrhagic bacteria
	Marked bandemia is associated with *Shigella*
Stool leukocytes	This test has an 80% positive predictive value for colitis
	An abnormal result is typically > 5/high power microscopic field
Stool culture	This rules out:
	• enterohemorrhagic *E. coli*
	◦ Order evaluation for strain O157:H7 (the most common bacterial cause of hemolytic-uremic syndrome) when culture results are positive for *E. coli*[8]
	• *Salmonella* (typhoid fever; handling poultry or reptiles such as turtles)
	• *Shigella* (dysentery)
	• *Campylobacter* (undercooked meat, unpasteurized milk)

ABOUT STOOL CULTURE

Note that stool culture has low sensitivity, particularly in samples obtained after the start of antibiotics: a negative result does not necessarily rule out bacterial enterocolitis. Repeat the test (up to several times over 1 week) if clinically suspected.

When stool culture cannot be performed within 2 hours of collection, refrigerate the sample (4°C, 39°F) or place it in transport medium.

OTHER TESTS

In severe cases with clinical compromise, use:

- ALP, ALT, GGT (and, as indicated, AST, direct and indirect bilirubin, PT/INR) to assess for ischemic or toxic liver damage
- BUN and creatinine/eGFR to assess renal function in patients with severe dehydration or hemodynamic compromise (shock)
- serum chemistries (electrolytes, glucose) and arterial blood gas (ABG) to assess acid-base status

In cases of suspected parasites or protozoans (e.g., *Entamoeba, Giardia*), use:

- stool microscopy for ova and parasites

When findings suggest protein-losing enteropathy in patients with enterohemorrhagic bacterial infections, use:

- serum albumin with consideration of fecal α_1-antitrypsin level

PEARLS

Do not eliminate *C. difficile* colitis from the clinical differential diagnosis just because the patient has not been on antibiotics: it may occur outside of this setting.

Immunocompromised patients may exhibit severe disease from organisms that usually cause clinically mild diarrhea (*Cryptosporidium, Cyclospora, Cystoisospora, Giardia*).

BLOODY DIARRHEA OR STOOL, CHRONIC

KEYS TO WORKUP

Bloody diarrhea of more than 2 to 4 weeks duration requires investigation.

Use laboratory testing to rule out infectious colitis. Note that symptoms and signs of infectious colitis may overlap with several other conditions, including celiac disease.

In addition, note that:

- There are no lab tests that can specifically diagnose inflammatory bowel disease (IBD). Laboratory studies may have value in assessing treatment response and monitoring for relapse.
- A diagnosis of Crohn disease comes from clinical history and specific signs on physical examination (e.g., anal fissures). Colonoscopic biopsy and histological evaluation confirm the diagnosis, and assess the severity and anatomic extent of disease.

LAB INVESTIGATIONS

TESTS FOR INITIAL WORKUP

- CBC: to assess the extent of inflammation
- stool culture: to exclude infectious bacterial etiologies
- stool WBC

SEROLOGIC TESTS FOR IBD

If IBD is suspected, tests such as perinuclear anti-neutrophil cytoplasmic antibody (p-ANCA) and anti-*Saccharomyces cerevisiae* antibody can prove helpful.

Note that serologic testing has insufficient sensitivity and specificity for screening and diagnosis of IBD, but may have promise in helping to distinguish among IBD subtypes.[9]

TESTS FOR MONITORING PATIENTS

Consider the following tests to manage (versus diagnose) chronic diarrhea:

- CRP, erythrocyte sedimentation rate (ESR), fecal calprotectin, and lactoferrin[10] (useful as biomarkers in monitoring disease for flares and response to treatment; note that ESR elevation is nonspecific)
- tests for nutritional markers (to evaluate malabsorption), including:
  - iron
  - ferritin
  - albumin
  - prealbumin (transthyretin)
  - vitamin B_{12}
  - folate
  - calcium
  - magnesium

DIARRHEA, WATERY, ACUTE

KEYS TO WORKUP

Watery diarrhea with abrupt onset and lasting less than 2 to 3 weeks typically implies disease in the small bowel and is usually due to infectious causes:

- viruses—e.g., rotavirus, adenovirus, calicivirus, astrovirus, norovirus
- enterotoxigenic bacteria—e.g., *E. coli* (most common), *Vibrio cholerae*, *Klebsiella*, and *Clostridium*

- bacterial toxins—e.g., *Clostridium difficile*
- parasites—e.g., *Cryptosporidium*, *Giardia*

Question patients carefully about foods recently consumed, recent antibiotic use, and places recently travelled: this may point to likely causative agents.

Note that patients may also present with low-grade fever and/or vomiting.

Clinical evidence is an important guide in decisions about antibiotic therapy. Laboratory testing can help establish causative bacteria or parasites, and (with bacterial sensitivity testing) can help tailor antibiotic therapy.

See also: vomiting, p. 93

LAB INVESTIGATIONS

STOOL CULTURE AND STOOL LEUKOCYTES
This combination of tests determines if an episode of acute diarrhea is invasive (e.g., enteroinvasive *E. coli*).

For stool leukocytes, a normal result is < 5/high power microscopic field.

Note that these tests are not useful predictors of stool culture positivity or response to treatment.[11]

OTHER STOOL TESTS

SUSPECTED ADENOVIRUS
Order:

- adenovirus enzyme immunoassay (EIA)

SUSPECTED ROTAVIRUS
Order either:

- rotavirus EIA
- rotavirus latex agglutination

SEVERE CASES WITH SIGNIFICANT HYPOVOLEMIA
OR CLINICAL COMPROMISE
Order:

- creatinine/eGFR to assess renal function
- ALP, ALT, GGT (and, as indicated, AST, direct and indirect bilirubin, PT/INR) to assess for ischemic liver damage
- serum chemistries (electrolytes, glucose) and ABG to assess acid-base status

HISTORY OF BACKPACKING OR
EXPOSURE TO ANIMALS
Consider:

- stool microscopy (O+P) to detect *Giardia*, *Cryptosporidium* or other parasitic cause of diarrhea
- *Giardia lamblia* cyst antigen assay: enzyme-linked immunosorbent assay (ELISA)
- polymerase chain reaction (PCR) testing for *Cryptosporidium* (not available in many labs; call your lab beforehand to discuss test availability)

RECENT HOSPITALIZATION
OR ANTIBIOTIC USE
Consider:

- antigen detection assay for *Clostridium difficile*: immunofluorescent assay (IFA), latex agglutination
  - Note: this test cannot distinguish between *C. difficile* colonization and infection.
- PCR assay for *Clostridium difficile* toxin B
- *C. difficile* toxin A, B, A+B (EIA)
  - Note: *C. difficile* toxin is very unstable and quickly degrades. Stool samples more than 2 hours old may yield false-negative results. Test promptly or refrigerate specimens to slow toxin degradation.

NOT USUALLY INDICATED

The following tests are not clinically indicated in most situations:

- stool pH: a result of < 5.5 suggests carbohydrate intolerance (seen with viral enteritis), but this is typically transient
- stool culture after the start of antibiotic treatment: this has a low clinical yield

DIARRHEA, WATERY, CHRONIC

KEYS TO WORKUP

The differential diagnosis of watery diarrhea, or loose stools for more than 3 weeks, is broad and includes:

- intestinal infections (bacterial and viral)
- eosinophilic gastroenteritis
- food allergy
- hyperthyroidism
- inflammatory bowel disease (Crohn disease and ulcerative colitis)
- irritable bowel syndrome
- food intolerance (e.g., lactose, sorbitol, Olestra, etc.)
- malabsorption syndromes (including pancreatic disorders such as chronic pancreatitis, pancreatic enzyme deficiencies, cystic fibrosis)
- medications (especially laxatives and antibiotics)
- microscopic colitis (lymphocytic colitis and collagenous colitis)
- parasite infestation
- ischemic colitis
- tumours
- immune-altered states (AIDS, other immune-deficient states, autoimmune diseases)

Clinical history is essential in narrowing the differential diagnosis. Clinical laboratory evaluation, often in conjunction with other workup including EGD and colonoscopy with biopsy evaluation, may help establish a diagnosis in cases where the diagnosis is not clear. Laboratory testing is not indicated in all cases, but should be tailored to the clinical differential diagnosis.

LAB INVESTIGATIONS

STOOL CULTURE

Reserve this test for cases where there is a strong clinical suspicion of bacterial infection, because stool culture has a low yield in watery diarrhea and when specimen collection occurs after the start of antibiotic therapy.

The low sensitivity of the test may make repeat testing necessary (several samples submitted over 1 week).

STOOL WBC

A normal result is < 5/high power microscopic field.

An elevated stool WBC count indicates colitis, which may be due to a variety of etiologies (infectious, inflammatory bowel disease, etc.).

In combination with stool culture, this test helps determine if an episode of acute diarrhea is due to an enteroinvasive organism (e.g., enteroinvasive *E. coli*).

Note that this test is not useful as a predictor of stool culture positivity or response to treatment.[11]

TESTS FOR HYPERTHYROIDISM

To rule out hyperthyroidism:

- Start by measuring thyroid-stimulating hormone (TSH), which is the single best initial test for thyroid disorders.
- Follow up with T_4 if the initial TSH is suppressed.

Note that T_3 is rarely indicated, and is useful only when TSH is suppressed but free T_4 is normal (a pattern known as T_3 toxicosis).

See: hyperthyroidism, p. 33

OTHER TESTS

Use the following tests as clinically warranted:

- CBC to look for eosinophilia in suspected cases of eosinophilic gastroenteritis
- fecal ova and parasites (*Giardia, Cryptosporidium, Cyclospora, Entamoeba histolytica,* microsporidia)
- fecal eosinophil count if parasite infestation is suspected

NOT RECOMMENDED

Generalized serum allergen testing (RAST) has a poor clinical yield for patients with suspected allergic gastroenteritis. Careful dietary history and patient monitoring of specific food intake are more helpful.

PEARLS

A history of immunocompromised status should prompt evaluation for opportunistic organisms (e.g., *Cryptosporidium, Cyclospora,* etc.).[12]

In many patients, a specific cause cannot be identified, and many of these patients may have irritable bowel syndrome (a diagnosis of exclusion). Colonoscopic biopsies may be helpful in establishing a diagnosis by ruling out other entities that can cause histologic abnormalities.

FREQUENT BOWEL MOVEMENTS

KEYS TO WORKUP

The clinical differential diagnosis for patients with frequent bowel movements includes malabsorptive, metabolic, and inflammatory bowel disorders, including:

- celiac disease
- Crohn disease
- hyperthyroidism
- irritable bowel syndrome
- ulcerative colitis
- medication-associated bowel frequency

Definitive diagnosis often rests on colonoscopy with biopsy.

Irritable bowel syndrome has nonspecific clinical and laboratory findings with normal endoscopy and is a diagnosis of exclusion.

When the cause is not obvious from clinical history and physical examination, lab testing may be helpful in narrowing the differential diagnosis.

LAB INVESTIGATIONS

CBC
Order this test as clinically indicated, to assess for inflammation and infection.

FIT AND gFOBT
Order a FIT or gFOBT as clinically indicated.

If positive, these may indicate GI bleeding, which may point to a more clinically serious cause of frequent bowel movements, such as ulcerative colitis.

See: FIT and gFOBT, p. 67

STOOL WBC
A normal result is < 5/high power microscopic field.

An elevated WBC count indicates colitis, which may be due to a variety of etiologies (infectious, inflammatory bowel disease, etc.).

In combination with stool culture, this test helps determine if an episode of acute diarrhea is due to an enteroinvasive organism (e.g., enteroinvasive *E. coli*).

Note that this test is not useful as a predictor of stool culture positivity or response to treatment.[11]

TESTS FOR HYPERTHYROIDISM
To rule out hyperthyroidism:

- Start with TSH, which is the single best initial test for thyroid disorders.
- Follow up with T_4 if the initial TSH is suppressed.

Note that T_3 is rarely indicated, and is useful only when TSH is suppressed but free T_4 is normal (a pattern known as T_3 toxicosis).

See: hyperthyroidism, p. 33

CELIAC DISEASE SEROLOGIES
Order the following tests if celiac disease is suspected:

- IgA tTG antibody (tTG)
- IgA antiendomysial antibody (EMA)
- total IgA level

See: celiac disease serologies, pp. 65–67

GI BLEEDING, ACUTE

KEYS TO WORKUP
Use laboratory testing primarily to assess:

- the degree of blood loss (CBC)
- whether any end-organ dysfunction is present due to hypoperfusion

Depending on comorbidities and the degree of blood loss, the severity of the clinical condition may warrant additional testing (e.g., acid-base studies including ABG, DIC workup, etc.).

LAB INVESTIGATIONS

CBC

This is a useful test in all cases to assess the degree of blood loss.

PT/INR, aPTT

Use these tests if findings suggest a coagulation disorder.

See: disorders of coagulation, p. 145

OTHER TESTS

Use the following tests to assess end-organ function as clinically indicated, and depending on the degree of blood loss:

- metabolic and electrolyte abnormalities: serum chemistries (BUN, creatinine, electrolytes, glucose)
- liver tests: ALP, ALT, AST, direct and indirect bilirubin, GGT, PT/INR
- renal function tests: creatinine/eGFR
- cardiac enzymes (troponin I or troponin T): for patients at risk of myocardial infarction (chest pain, dyspnea, elderly, history of coronary artery disease)

PEARLS

DISTINGUISHING ACUTE BLEEDING

CBC may initially not reflect the degree of blood loss (Hb and Hct may be normal, or at the patient's baseline, initially) since the patient is losing whole blood.

Patients with acute bleeding have normocytic RBCs (normal MCV). Patients with iron-deficiency anemia or anemia of chronic disease have microcytic RBCs (low MCV) with anisocytosis (increased RDW). Note that acute GI bleeding and chronic anemia commonly coexist.

ABOUT RENAL FUNCTION TESTS

Elevated BUN/creatinine ratio (> 20:1) is more commonly seen in upper GI bleeding (as opposed to lower GI bleeding), and implies dehydration and decreased renal perfusion.

Rising creatinine indicates acute renal failure, which may be secondary to renal hypoperfusion (as seen in shock or hemodynamic compromise).

Note that the following combination of tests can be used to monitor renal status in hospitalized patients with compromised hemodynamic function (particularly patients requiring aggressive management including vasopressor support):

- serial BUN and creatinine measurement
- urine output measurement

JAUNDICE

KEYS TO WORKUP

Jaundice is a yellowish staining of the mucous membranes, sclera, and skin by bilirubin. Typically, jaundice occurs after serum bilirubin rises above about 50 μmol/L (2.5 mg/dL).

PREHEPATIC, INTRAHEPATIC, AND POSTHEPATIC CAUSES

Dysfunction of any of the 3 phases in bilirubin metabolism may lead to jaundice:

- prehepatic: most bilirubin is produced from metabolism of heme (from the breakdown of RBCs), with a lesser amount of heme produced from the breakdown of muscle myoglobin and cytochromes, or from ineffective erythropoiesis; bilirubin enters the liver via the circulation (plasma) for conjugation and excretion
- intrahepatic: within the hepatocyte, bilirubin is enzymatically conjugated to glucuronide,

making it soluble in bile; dysfunction is caused by enzymatic disorders of bilirubin metabolism
- posthepatic: bile (stored in the gallbladder) is transported through biliary and cystic ducts to the ampulla and into the duodenal lumen

UNCONJUGATED VERSUS CONJUGATED CAUSES

Causes of unconjugated hyperbilirubinemia include:

- drugs causing hemolysis, hemolytic anemia, hemoglobinopathies, Gilbert syndrome (enzymatic disorder)
- large hematomas (occasionally)

Causes of conjugated hyperbilirubinemia include:

- intrahepatic:
  - viruses
  - alcohol
  - autoimmune: primary sclerosing cholangitis (PSC); primary biliary cirrhosis (PBC); autoimmune hepatitis
  - drugs causing cholestasis, enzyme disorders (rare)
- posthepatic: intrinsic or extrinsic obstruction of bile duct system (gallstones, biliary tract tumours, pancreatitis, cholangitis)

GUIDES TO LABORATORY INVESTIGATIONS

Make decisions about laboratory investigations based on:

- clinical history
  - acholic stools
  - travel history (e.g., to areas where HAV and HBV are endemic)
  - factors associated with viral hepatitis (exposure to body fluids, intravenous drug use, etc.)

- ° acuity of onset
- ° medications
- ° prior or current medical diagnoses
- ° surgical history
- ° associated abdominal pain, with severity

- physical findings
  - ° signs of cirrhosis or portal hypertension
  - ° hepatomegaly

LAB INVESTIGATIONS

Order tests as clinically indicated (see the breakdown that follows).

Test	Significance
ALP and GGT	Elevated in cholestasis
ALT and AST	Markers of hepatocellular injury
	Levels > 1500 U/L typically indicate acute liver injury from drugs or ischemia
Autoimmune hepatobiliary markers	
• AMA	Positive in almost all PBC patients
• ANA	Typically positive in autoimmune hepatitis
• ALKM-1	Positive in autoimmune hepatitis type II (typically female children and teenagers, often severe disease)
• ASMA	Positive in autoimmune hepatitis and in 20%–50% of PSC patients, but not specific
• p-ANCA	Positive in 80% of PSC patients, but not specific
• quantitative immunoglobulins	Typically elevated total immunoglobulin or IgG fraction in autoimmune hepatitis (1.5 X normal)
CBC	Useful in detecting anemia
Indirect and direct bilirubin	Distinguishes prehepatic, intrahepatic, and posthepatic causes of jaundice
Liver biopsy	May be helpful in the workup of jaundice when clinically warranted, particularly in diagnosing biliary tract disorders (PSC or PBC) and autoimmune hepatitis

Continued on p. 89

Continued from p. 88

Peripheral blood smear and reticulocyte count	
• peripheral blood smear	Identifies reticulocytes and schistocytes in the workup of hemolysis
• reticulocyte count	Identifies marrow response to anemia
PT/INR	Marker of severe acute liver injury
	Typically seen with ischemia or drug toxicity, and possibly in jaundice with end-stage liver failure
	Note: iatrogenic causes of elevated PT/INR must be excluded (e.g., Coumadin/warfarin)
Urinalysis	Detects semiquantitative bilirubin level and the presence of blood and/or hemoglobin in urine
	Urine bilirubin is typically elevated in conjugated hyperbilirubinemia, and not elevated in unconjugated hyperbilirubinemia
Viral hepatitis markers*	Identify particular viral etiologies
• hepatitis A virus IgM antibody (anti-HAV IgM)*	
• HAV, total antibody	
• hepatitis B core antibody (anti-HBcAb, IgG, and IgM)*	
• hepatitis B surface antigen (HBsAg)	
• hepatitis B surface antibody (anti-HBsAb)	
• hepatitis C antibody (anti-HCV)	
• HIV (in at-risk populations, to rule out HIV cholangiopathy)	

*NOTES:

• Hepatitis B e antigen (HBeAg) and hepatitis B e antibody (anti-HBeAb) are **not** recommended in the initial laboratory workup of suspected viral hepatitis; rather, they are used to assess HBV disease severity or for treatment eligibility and/or monitoring.
• Hepatitis E virus (HEV) is not endemic to Canada or the US, so test for HEV (serology for anti-HEV antibodies) only if the patient has travelled to, or has had contact with persons from, countries where HEV is endemic.
• Given the low prevalence of HAV infection in Canada, many positive results for anti-HAV IgM may be false. Clinical correlation is required.
• Anti-HBc IgM is frequently not included in viral hepatitis testing protocols because there is usually no window between disappearance of HBsAg and serologic evidence of resolved infection.

PEARLS

PSEUDOJAUNDICE

Pseudojaundice can occur in patients with a high intake of vegetables high in beta-carotene (e.g., carrots, melons, squash). Pseudojaundice presents with no scleral icterus on physical examination and normal serum bilirubin (and other lab tests).

PAINLESS JAUNDICE IN OLDER PATIENTS

For older patients with painless jaundice, always consider bile duct obstruction by malignancy in the clinical diagnosis.

Laboratory testing in this setting is not diagnostic in and of itself. Radiologic correlation (i.e., ultrasound, CT with guided biopsy, or cholangiography) and endoscopy (ERCP with brushing cytology or biopsy) are crucial to establishing a diagnosis.

PREVALENCE OF HAV, HBV, HCV

Hepatitis A, B, and C account for about 90% of cases of acute hepatitis in Canada.[13] Autoimmune hepatitis has an incidence of 1 to 2 per 100 000 per year, and a prevalence of 10 to 20 per 100 000. Therefore, the following 2-step approach could save money:

- perform the viral hepatitis panel first (to rule out the more common disease group)
- follow up with an autoimmune hepatitis panel in patients whose viral hepatitis panel is negative

MALODOROUS STOOL

KEYS TO WORKUP

Malodorous stools are typically pale and bulky, and often coincident with flatulence. They typically signal fat malabsorption.

Depending on clinical evidence, testing is useful to rule out:

- *Giardia* enteritis
- malabsorption syndromes

Chronic malabsorption presents with:

- weight loss (most common sign)

It may also present with:

- hypoalbuminemia in more pronounced cases which, if severe, will lead to ascites
- macrocytic anemia if vitamin B_{12} or folate deficiency is present; or microcytic anemia if iron deficiency is present
- secondary hyperparathyroidism from malabsorption of calcium with resultant deficiency
- bone mineralization disorders from decreased absorption of fat-soluble vitamin D
- clotting disorders from decreased absorption of fat-soluble vitamin K

Laboratory testing helps gauge the clinical severity of malabsorption, but is not as helpful in arriving at an etiology (with the exception of celiac disease serologies).

LAB INVESTIGATIONS

SUSPECTED *GIARDIA*

If the patient has a history of backpacking or exposure to animals, consider ordering:

- stool microscopy (O+P) to detect *Giardia*
- *Giardia lamblia* cyst antigen assay: ELISA

TESTS FOR MALABSORPTION

If a malabsorption syndrome is suspected, use the following panel of tests to gauge its severity and help in establishing the etiology (see the breakdown that follows).

Test	Notes
CBC	WBC is typically elevated in inflammation or infection
	Hb and Hct may be low in anemia due to protein, mineral and/or vitamin malabsorption
Ferritin	Low levels of ferritin may point to iron deficiency, which in turn may arise through malabsorption of dietary iron
Folate and vitamin B_{12}	Decreased levels due to malabsorption may result in macrocytic anemia and/or other abnormalities
Serum chemistries (BUN, creatinine, electrolytes, glucose)	Serum chemistries may be abnormal in chronic malabsorptive syndromes, but are not diagnostic per se
Calcium and magnesium	Calcium and magnesium may be deficient in malabsorptive syndromes
Albumin	Albumin evaluates the degree of protein deficiency due to malabsorption
Fecal elastase and chymotrypsin (pancreatic enzymes)	These distinguish between pancreatic and intestinal malabsorption, but note that fecal elastase is not an accurate marker of pancreatic steatorrhea[14]
Serum IgA, quantitative	This rules out IgA deficiency, which is often associated with malabsorptive syndromes
	Note: IgA deficiency gives false-negative IgA tTG antibody results (because the IgA tTG antibody fraction is the typical testing target)
IgA tTG antibody (tTG) IgA antiendomysial antibody (EMA) Total IgA level *See: celiac disease serologies, pp. 65–67*	These rule out celiac disease
Fecal fat quantitation	This checks for poor absorption of dietary fat (typically requires 72-hour stool sample)

PEARLS

Esophagogastroduodenoscopy (EGD) with mucosal biopsy can help evaluate causes of malabsorption, such as celiac disease and Whipple disease.

Cystic fibrosis, another cause of malabsorption, is usually diagnosed on clinical grounds, although sweat chloride testing and mutation analysis testing may help.

VOMITING

KEYS TO WORKUP

The diagnosis of vomiting typically comes from clinical signs and symptoms (e.g., viral or bacterial gastroenteritis; endotoxin-associated food poisoning; overdose or drug toxicity). For chronic vomiting, clinical history may reveal a chronic metabolic disorder as the etiology (e.g., diabetic ketoacidosis).

Laboratory testing usually has little or no role in the diagnosis of vomiting. It can help manage vomiting (particularly severe vomiting) in assessing:

- dehydration
- acid-base status (in more severe or prolonged cases, loss of hydrochloric acid through prolonged vomiting may occasionally result in dehydration and metabolic alkalosis, particularly in debilitated patients who may not be able to compensate for the acid-base disturbance)

The value of other testing depends on the etiology or on coexisting signs—for example, jaundice, head trauma, or mental status changes (radiologic workup has far greater importance in neurologic-associated vomiting).

Red flags for urgent additional testing (laboratory and otherwise) include:

- distended abdomen
- headache, stiff neck, or mental status change
- signs of hypovolemia
- peritoneal signs

LAB INVESTIGATIONS

When clinically warranted, the following panels of tests can help determine how to manage vomiting (see the breakdown that follows).

Clinical scenario	Test panel
Obtunded patients or patients with prolonged severe vomiting	ABG to assess acid-base status
	CBC to assess Hb and Hct for anemia and WBC for possibility of infection
	Serum chemistries (BUN, creatinine, electrolytes, glucose) to assess for electrolyte imbalances, possible acid-base disturbance
	Serum ketones and glucose to evaluate for metabolic abnormalities such as diabetic ketoacidosis (DKA)
	BUN and creatinine/eGFR to evaluate renal function and for dehydration
Patients with vomiting and jaundice	Liver function tests: ALP, ALT, AST, direct and indirect bilirubin, GGT, PT/INR
	If liver tests are elevated, consider a viral hepatitis panel

PEARLS

In any reproductive-age female with vomiting, always rule out pregnancy-associated vomiting (hyperemesis gravidarum) with quantitative serum β-hCG or qualitative urine β-hCG.

Petechiae on the face and torso may occur with forceful vomiting. In an otherwise well-appearing patient, unless there is clinical suspicion, this should not prompt a laboratory workup for coagulopathy or thrombocytopenia.

Consider infectious etiology, especially when vomiting and diarrhea occur simultaneously (*see: acute bloody diarrhea, p. 74, and acute watery diarrhea, p. 77*).

WEIGHT LOSS, UNEXPLAINED

KEYS TO WORKUP

Clinical history and physical exam prove helpful in the majority of diagnoses of unexplained weight loss. Laboratory testing may help primarily in ruling out metabolic causes.

The leading causes of unintentional weight loss are:

- depression
- cancer
- cardiac disorders
- benign GI diseases

Medications and hyperthyroidism are additional causes.

A specific cause cannot be identified in one-quarter of elderly patients.

LAB INVESTIGATIONS

FIT AND gFOBT

Order a FIT or gFOBT to screen for colonic carcinoma.

See: FIT and gFOBT, p. 67

TESTS FOR HYPERTHYROIDISM

To rule out hyperthyroidism:

- Start with TSH, which is the single best initial test for thyroid disorders.
- Follow up with T_4 if the initial TSH is suppressed.

Note that T_3 is rarely indicated, and is useful only when TSH is suppressed but free T_4 is normal (a pattern known as T_3 toxicosis).

See: hyperthyroidism, p. 33

URINALYSIS

This helps to rule out infection and renal dysfunction.

SERUM ALBUMIN AND PREALBUMIN (TRANSTHYRETIN)

These tests evaluate possible malnutrition.

PEARLS

Carcinoembryonic antigen (CEA) is useful in monitoring for the recurrence of colorectal carcinoma (sensitivity around 80%), especially in detection of liver metastasis, but is not recommended to screen for, or diagnose, occult colorectal cancer. The sensitivity of CEA for detecting early-stage (Dukes A and B) colorectal cancer is only 36% with a reference value of 2.5 μg/L (2.5 ng/mL); CEA is not specific for colorectal carcinoma and may be elevated in most types of advanced adenocarcinomas.[15]

REFERENCES

1   Cartwright SL, Knudson MP. Evaluation of acute abdominal pain in adults. *Am Fam Physician*. 2008;77(7):971–978. Medline:18441863

2   Hill ID, Dirks MH, Liptak GS, et al, and the North American Society for Pediatric Gastroenterology, Hepatology and Nutrition. Guideline for the diagnosis and treatment of celiac disease in children: recommendations of the North American Society for Pediatric Gastroenterology, Hepatology and Nutrition. *J Pediatr Gastroenterol Nutr*. 2005;40(1):1–19. http://dx.doi.org/10.1097/00005176-200501000-00001. Medline:15625418

3   Kagnoff MF, and the AGA Institute. AGA Institute medical position statement on the diagnosis and management of celiac disease. *Gastroenterology*. 2006;131(6):1977–1980. http://dx.doi.org/10.1053/j.gastro.2006.10.003. Medline:17087935

4   Bai J, Zeballos E, Fried GR, et al. WGO-OMGE practice guideline: celiac disease. http://www.worldgastroenterology.org/global-guidelines.html February 2005. Accessed November 22, 2013.

5   Browning JD, Horton JD. Gallstone disease and its complications. *Semin Gastrointest Dis*. 2003;14(4):165–177. Medline:14719767

6   Guidelines and Protocols Advisory Committee, British Columbia Medical Association and British Columbia Ministry of Health Services. Viral Hepatitis Testing. http://www.bcguidelines.ca/pdf/vihep.pdf. January 1, 2012. Accessed November 21, 2013.

7   Runyon BA. Refractory ascites. *Semin Liver Dis*. 1993;13(4):343–351. http://dx.doi.org/10.1055/s-2007-1007362. Medline:8303315

8   Holtz LR, Neill MA, Tarr PI. Acute bloody diarrhea: a medical emergency for patients of all ages. *Gastroenterology*. 2009;136(6):1887–1898. http://dx.doi.org/10.1053/j.gastro.2009.02.059. Medline:19457417

9   Wong A, Bass D. Laboratory evaluation of inflammatory bowel disease. *Curr Opin Pediatr*. 2008;20(5):566–570. http://dx.doi.org/10.1097/MOP.0b013e32830d3aaf. Medline:18781120

10 Abraham BP, Kane S. Fecal markers: calprotectin and lactoferrin. *Gastroenterol Clin North Am*. 2012;41(2):483–495. http://dx.doi.org/10.1016/j.gtc.2012.01.007. Medline:22500530

11 Herbert ME. Medical myth: Measuring white blood cells in the stools is useful in the management of acute diarrhea. *West J Med*. 2000;172(6):414. http://dx.doi.org/10.1136/ewjm.172.6.414. Medline:10854401

12 Krones E, Högenauer C. Diarrhea in the immunocompromised patient. *Gastroenterol Clin North Am*. 2012;41(3):677–701. http://dx.doi.org/10.1016/j.gtc.2012.06.009. Medline:22917171

13 Health Canada. Hepatitis. http://www.hc-sc.gc.ca/hc-ps/dc-ma/hep-eng.php. Updated July 8, 2008. Accessed October 18, 2013.

14 DiMagno MJ, DiMagno EP. Chronic pancreatitis. *Curr Opin Gastroenterol*. 2010;26(5):490–498. http://dx.doi.org/10.1097/MOG.0b013e32833d11b2. Medline:20693896

15 Duffy MJ. Carcinoembryonic antigen as a marker for colorectal cancer: is it clinically useful? *Clin Chem*. 2001;47(4):624–630. Medline:11274010

Genitourinary system

Dr. Davinder Sidhu

ABBREVIATIONS

ABG	arterial blood gas	HSV	herpes simplex virus
ADH	antidiuretic hormone	IgA	immunoglobulin A
ALP	alkaline phosphatase	IV	intravenous
ALT	alanine aminotransferase	LE	leukocyte esterase
ARF	acute renal failure	MGUS	monoclonal gammopathy
AST	aspartate aminotransferase	PSA	prostate-specific antigen
BPH	benign prostatic hyperplasia	PT/INR	prothrombin time or international
CHF	congestive heart failure		normalized ratio
CML	chronic myelocytic leukemia	PTH	parathyroid hormone
CMML	chronic myelomonocytic	RBC	red blood cell
	leukemia	RTA	renal tubular acidosis
CRF	chronic renal failure	SIADH	syndrome of inappropriate
DI	diabetes insipidus		antidiuretic hormone
DIC	disseminated intravascular		secretion
	coagulation	SLE	systemic lupus erythematosus
eGFR	estimated glomerular filtration	SSRI	selective serotonin reuptake
	rate		inhibitor
GBM	glomerular basement membrane	STD	sexually transmitted disease
GFR	glomerular filtration rate	TSH	thyroid-stimulating hormone
GGT	γ-glutamyltransferase		(thyrotropin)
GI	gastrointestinal	TTKG	transtubular potassium gradient
GU	genitourinary	UTI	urinary tract infection
HPF	high power microscopic field	WBC	white blood cell

OVERALL APPROACH

Prerenal, renal, postrenal dysfunction

Most clinical genitourinary (GU) presentations can be divided into prerenal, renal, and postrenal causes similar to the diagnostic approach used in acute and chronic renal dysfunction.

For GU dysfunction:

- prerenal causes can include systemic diseases such as diabetes, medications, and issues with hypertension or renal perfusion
- renal causes may be implicated in hematuria, electrolyte imbalances, and acid-base disturbances
- postrenal issues can contribute to dysuria, increased urinary frequency, and incontinence

Infections and infectious sequelae can be implicated at any site in the GU tract.

Findings in urine

Urinalysis requires direct examination of urine and provides key information about GU system function (see the breakdown that follows). Note that values outside of the reference range are important, as small numbers of RBC, WBC, and hyaline casts can be seen in normal urine.

Findings in urine	Significance
Casts (clumps of cells formed in the tubules)	
• fatty urine casts	May indicate nephritic syndrome, SLE, ethylene glycol poisoning, or mercury toxicity
• hyaline casts	High numbers of casts may be seen in the context of proteinuria
	Low numbers of casts have no clinical significance
• RBC casts	Can indicate serious kidney disorders including acute glomerulonephritis and SLE nephritis

Continued on p. 101

Continued from p. 100

• renal tubular epithelial cell casts	Indicate damage to the tubules (from renal tubular necrosis, transplant rejection, or viral disease)
• urine waxy casts	Indicate acute renal disease, malignant hypertension, or diabetic nephropathy
• WBC and RBC casts	Generally indicate upper urinary tract infection (UTI)
Crystals	Indicate renal stones or metabolic disorders
Leukocyte esterase (LE), nitrite, and WBCs	Indicate UTI
Protein	Indicates impaired renal function
Abnormal specific gravity	
• high specific gravity	Indicates concentrated urine (volume depletion)
• low specific gravity	Indicates dilute urine May reflect impaired ability of the kidneys to concentrate urine

Normal ranges for GU function

The following tables will help you interpret laboratory findings from tests in this section.

Table 7. Urinalysis, normal values

Characteristic	Normal finding
Appearance and colour	Clear or yellow, straw
Crystals	Few or negative
Glucose	Negative
Ketones	Negative
LE	Negative
Nitrite	Negative
pH	4.6–8.0
Protein	2–8 mg/dL (10–150 mg/24 h)
RBC casts	Negative
RBCs	1–2/HPF
Specific gravity	1.005–1.030
WBC casts	Negative
WBCs	3–4/HPF

Table 8. Normal values for urine electrolytes

Urine electrolytes	Reference ranges
Calcium	Male: < 6.8 mmol/day (< 275 mg/day) Female: < 6.2 mmol/day (< 250 mg/day)
Chloride	110–250 mmol/day (110–250 mEq/day)
Magnesium	3–4.3 mmol/day (< 150 mg/day)
Phosphorus	29–42 mmol/day (900–1300 mg/day)
Potassium	40–80 mmol/day (40–80 mEq/day)
Sodium	30–280 mmol/day (30–280 mEq/day)

DISORDERS AND CLINICAL PRESENTATIONS

DYSURIA

KEYS TO WORKUP

Dysuria, or pain and discomfort during urination, is most frequently caused by urinary tract infection, but other causes exist.

Laboratory tests such as urinalysis and urine culture can help to determine the presence of infection and confirm a suspected diagnosis. Laboratory testing can also help rule in and rule out other causes, including calculi, hypoestrogenism, interstitial cystitis, neoplasm, noninfectious inflammation, trauma, and psychogenic disorders.

Patients with dysuria fall into 2 categories:

- with pyuria (leukocytes on microscopy, positive nitrite and/or LE)
- without pyuria (no leukocytes on microscopy, negative nitrite and LE)

Dysuria without pyuria can be caused by:

- interstitial cystitis
- systemic causes such as estrogen deficiency
- urethritis (*Candida*, HSV)
- vaginitis (*Candida*, *Gardnerella*, carcinoma)

Patients with dysuria and pyuria can further present with or without hematuria:

- dysuria with pyuria, hematuria, and bacteria suggests:
  - upper urinary tract infection or pyelonephritis, especially if WBC casts are present
  - lower urinary tract infection or cystitis if WBC clumps are present
- dysuria with pyuria, but no hematuria or no bacteria (nitrite negative), suggests infection from:
  - *Chlamydia*
  - gonococcus
  - *Trichomonas*

LAB INVESTIGATIONS

URINALYSIS
Begin with this test (see Table 7 for normal urinalysis values).

OTHER TESTS
Base decisions about other tests on the clinical situation.

In sexually active individuals, consider testing for STDs (*Chlamydia*, gonococcus, or *Trichomonas*).

HEMATURIA

KEYS TO WORKUP
Make decisions about laboratory testing based on clinical presentation and patient characteristics.

Infection is the most common cause of hematuria in some younger women, but also consider other causes, particularly in older individuals or in the presence of other symptoms. Blood contamination of urine by menstruation or lower GI source (e.g., hemorrhoids) may occur: careful patient questioning is important to exclude these possibilities.

Note that apparent hematuria can arise from myoglobinuria or red supernatant in urine due to natural dyes found in some foods (beets).

Microscopic examination for RBCs is the best screening exam and can determine the cause of true hematuria as either:

- extraglomerular (isomorphic RBCs with no casts)
- glomerular (dysmorphic RBCs with or without RBC casts)

Extraglomerular causes include:

- UTI
- tumours, calculi, and cysts in the upper urinary tract
- tumours, trauma, calculi, or benign prostatic hyperplasia (BPH) in the lower urinary tract
  Note that microhematuria may sometimes be present without apparent cause. For glomerular causes of hematuria, see the breakdown that follows.

Findings in urine	Possible glomerular etiology
Active sediment, no protein	Anti–glomerular basement membrane (GBM) antibodies
	Immune-complex deposition (poststreptococcal infection, lupus, and IgA nephropathy)
	Pauci-immune disease (Wegener)
Benign sediment, no protein	IgA nephropathy
	Thin GBM disease
	Alport disease
Active sediment, protein	Membranoproliferative glomerulonephritis
	Lupus glomerulonephritis
	Postinfectious glomerulonephritis

LAB INVESTIGATIONS

URINE MICROSCOPY

This is the best screening exam for hematuria and should be part of your initial workup.

This test identifies cells, casts, and crystals.

Order follow-up tests of urine culture and antibiotic sensitivity:

- if urinalysis and/or microscopy suggest UTI (pyuria with or without nitrite or bacteria)
- if UTI is suspected clinically

URINALYSIS

Order this test as part of your initial workup. It assesses bacterial nitrite (e.g., gram-negative bacteria), leukocyte esterase, protein, and specific gravity (see Table 7 for normal urinalysis values).

OTHER TESTS

Select other tests depending on the clinical situation:

- urine myoglobin: this excludes systemic causes (e.g., malignant hyperthermia, rhabdomyolysis, skeletal or cardiac muscle ischemia, trauma)
- urine cystine and uric acid levels: use this to assess patients with renal calculus formation and identify patients at risk for stone formation
- urine protein electrophoresis and immunofixation: use this to identify immunoglobulin proteins (suggestive of autoimmune disease if polyclonal; indicative of MGUS or plasma cell dyscrasia if monoclonal)
- prostate-specific antigen (PSA) levels: consider this in the case of older males with BPH-like urinary obstructive symptoms to rule out carcinoma (note that other conditions, such

as prostatitis, can also produce elevated PSA levels)
- serum complement C3 and C4 levels: decreased levels are associated with disseminated intravascular coagulation (DIC), glomerulonephritis, gram-negative sepsis, and systemic lupus erythematosus (SLE)

HYPERKALEMIA

KEYS TO WORKUP

Laboratory testing for hyperkalemia should always include a serum creatinine level. Clinical history and patient presentation should guide decisions about further testing.

Hyperkalemia is commonly associated with either:

- renal failure (acute or chronic)
- use of potassium-sparing diuretics

It is usually defined as serum potassium > 5.5 mmol/L (> 5.5 mEq/L).

It can be due to 3 principal causes:

- reduced excretion, which can be due to:
  - decreased glomerular filtration rate from acute renal failure (ARF) or chronic renal failure (CRF)
  - factors affecting principal cell function (TTKG < 7 signals potassium-sparing diuretics, adrenal insufficiency, rhabdomyolysis, or diabetic nephropathy)
  - reduced flow through the distal nephron (TTKG > 7 signals congestive heart failure or hypotension)
- increased intake, which is typically secondary to IV potassium in the setting of reduced renal excretion

- intracellular shift, which can be due to:
  - ○ decreased entry of K^+ into cells (insulin deficiency or resistance, beta-2-blockade, alpha-1-stimulation, digoxin)
  - ○ excessive release of K^+ from cells (from non–anion gap metabolic acidosis exchange for H^+, hyperosmolarity, cell lysis)

LAB INVESTIGATIONS

SERUM CREATININE
Always order this test in cases of hyperkalemia.

ABG
Order an arterial blood gas (ABG) test as clinically indicated.

ABG assesses pH, bicarbonate, and CO_2 levels, which can affect electrolyte levels.

SERUM ELECTROLYTES
Order this test as clinically indicated to:

- detect shifts in electrolytes that can occur with pH changes and changes in serum osmolarity
- assess anion gap

ECG
Order this test if you suspect cardiac toxicity.

Results of concern include peaked T wave or widened QRS complex.

SERUM ALDOSTERONE AND PLASMA RENIN
Order these tests as clinically indicated.

Aldosterone is a potent mineralocorticoid that regulates sodium, potassium, and water balance.

In combination, these tests distinguish between primary and secondary (more common) hyperaldosteronism.

URINE DRUG AND TOXICOLOGY SCREEN

Order this test as clinically indicated to identify the causes of acidosis.

PEARLS

Any diagnosis of hyperkalemia must first exclude artifactual pseudohyperkalemia due to hemolysis, leukocytosis (CML, CMML), or in-vitro clot formation (thrombocytosis) in the collected specimen.

HYPOKALEMIA

KEYS TO WORKUP

Clinical history and patient presentation should guide decisions about laboratory testing for hypokalemia.

Hypokalemia is defined as serum potassium < 3.5 mmol/L (< 3.5 mEq/L).

It can be due to 3 primary causes:

- increased loss (most common)
- decreased intake (very rare)
- intracellular shift

Increased K^+ losses can be due to:

- gastrointestinal losses (TTKG < 4) due to:
  - diarrhea
  - vomiting
  - nasogastric suction
- renal losses (TTKG > 4) due to:
  - loop diuretics or Bartter syndrome
  - thiazide diuretics or Gitelman syndrome
  - magnesium depletion
  - antibiotics (carbenicillin, amphotericin B)
  - renal tubular acidosis (RTA) types 1 and 2
  - hyperaldosteronism or mineralocorticoid excess

- renal losses secondary to:
  - renal artery stenosis (hyperreninism)
  - Cushing syndrome
  - congenital adrenal hyperplasia
  - excessive licorice ingestion

Intracellular shifts of K^+ from serum into cells can be caused by:

- alkalemia (exchange of serum K^+ for intracellular H^+)
- refeeding syndrome
- insulin
- increased RBC production

LAB INVESTIGATIONS

ABG
Order this test as clinically indicated.

ABG assesses pH, bicarbonate, and CO_2 levels, which can affect electrolyte levels.

SERUM ELECTROLYTES
Order this test as clinically indicated to:

- detect shifts in electrolytes that can occur with pH changes and changes in serum osmolarity
- assess anion gap

SERUM ALDOSTERONE AND PLASMA RENIN
Order these tests as clinically indicated.

Aldosterone is a potent mineralocorticoid that regulates sodium, potassium, and water balance.

In combination, these tests distinguish between primary and secondary (more common) hyperaldosteronism.

URINE ALDOSTERONE ON 24-HOUR URINE COLLECTION
Order this test as clinically indicated.

This test is helpful in distinguishing primary and secondary (more common) hyperaldosteronism.

Low urine chloride distinguishes gastrointestinal loss from renal loss in volume-depleted individuals.

URINE ELECTROLYTES ON 24-HOUR URINE COLLECTION

Order this test as clinically indicated (see Table 8 for normal urine electrolyte values).

This test can distinguish causes of loss:

- $Urine_K$ < 30 mmol/day (30 mEq/day) suggests gastrointestinal (GI) losses.
- $Urine_K$ > 30 mmol/day (30 mEq/day) suggests renal losses.

HYPERNATREMIA

KEYS TO WORKUP

Sodium levels are critical to appropriate body fluid distribution, maintenance of osmotic pressure, acid-base balance, neurotransmitter function, and electrolyte balance within cells. Changes in serum sodium levels can have multiple clinical effects, which appropriate laboratory testing can distinguish.

Hypernatremia is defined as serum sodium > 145 mmol/L (> 145 mEq/L).

Causes include:

- excessive sodium intake
- excessive water deficits or dehydration (more common)

Sodium excess can be due to:

- increased intake (hypertonic saline or sodium bicarbonate ingestion)
- increased resorption (primary hyperaldosteronism)

Dehydration can result from:

- water losses, including:
  - renal losses (osmotic diuresis, diabetes insipidus)
  - GI losses (diarrhea)
  - insensible losses (burns, fever, exercise)
- inadequate intake (increased urine osmolality with decreased urine output)

LAB INVESTIGATIONS

URINE AND SERUM ELECTROLYTES
Order these tests as part of your initial workup (see Table 8 for normal urine electrolyte values).

ABG
Order this test as part of your initial workup.

This test assesses pH, bicarbonate, and CO_2 levels, which can affect electrolyte levels.

SERUM ALDOSTERONE AND PLASMA RENIN
Order these tests as clinically indicated.

Aldosterone is a potent mineralocorticoid that regulates sodium, potassium, and water balance.

In combination, these tests distinguish between primary and secondary (more common) hyperaldosteronism.

ADH SUPPRESSION
Test antidiuretic hormone (ADH) suppression as clinically indicated.

ADH controls the amount of water reabsorbed by the kidney:

- Inadequate ADH secretion results in diabetes insipidus (DI).
- Excess ADH secretion (often related to cancer—e.g., lung, pancreas, urinary tract,

hematopoetic) results in syndrome of inappropriate ADH (SIADH).

URINE OSMOLALITY

Order this test as clinically indicated.

Urine osmolality by random, timed, or 24-hour urine collection assesses:

- electrolyte and fluid balance
- the kidneys' ability to concentrate urine
- renal disease
- DI
- SIADH

Note that determination of both urine and serum osmolality aids in interpretation of results.

HYPONATREMIA

KEYS TO WORKUP

Diagnosis of hyponatremia requires exclusion of artifactual causes (pseudohyponatremia), including hyperglycemia, mannitol administration, hypertriglyceridemia, and paraproteinemia. Urine and serum osmolality and electrolytes differentiate between renal and extrarenal causes. Hypothyroidism should also be considered. Clinical history and patient presentation should guide decisions about further laboratory testing.

Hyponatremia is defined as serum sodium < 135 mmol/L (< 135 mEq/L) and considered severe when < 120 mmol/L (< 120 mEq/L).

Hyponatremia is caused by changes in water excretion ability. Individuals with intact water excretion can develop hyponatremia:

- due to excessive intake (polydipsia)
- due to medications with ADH-like or vasopressin-like effects (desmopressin, SSRIs, tricyclic antidepressants)

- secondary to malnutrition (low osmole intake or beer potomania)

Individuals with impaired water excretion develop hyponatremia:

- due to impaired desalination (Bartter or Gitelman syndromes, diuretic use)
- due to decreased GFR < 20 mL/min/1.73 m^2 (acute or chronic renal failure)
- secondary to SIADH (postoperation, neurologic trauma, drugs, malignancy)

Individuals with decreased effective arterial blood volume with appropriate ADH secretion to expand blood volume can also develop hyponatremia, particularly if they have:

- ongoing losses (renal losses, GI losses, bleeding)
- hypervolemia with large fluid volume shifts (CHF, cirrhosis, nephrotic syndrome, hypothyroidism, adrenal insufficiency, pregnancy)

LAB INVESTIGATIONS

URINE ELECTROLYTES

Order this test as part of your initial workup (see Table 8 for normal urine electrolyte values).

- Urine$_{Na}$ > 30 mmol/L (> 30 mEq/L) signals renal loss.
- Urine$_{Na}$ < 30 mmol/L (< 30 mEq/L) signals extrarenal loss.

URINE AND SERUM OSMOLALITY

Order these tests as part of your initial workup.

They assess:

- DI
- electrolyte and fluid balance
- the kidneys' ability to concentrate urine

- renal disease
- SIADH

ADH SUPPRESSION

Order this test as clinically indicated.

ADH controls the amount of water reabsorbed by the kidney.

- Inadequate ADH secretion results in DI.
- Excess ADH secretion (often related to cancer—e.g., lung, pancreas, urinary tract, hematopoietic) results in SIADH.

LIVER FUNCTION TESTS

Order these tests as clinically indicated (ALT, ALP, AST, indirect and direct bilirubin, GGT, PT/INR).

RENAL FUNCTION TESTS

Order these tests as clinically indicated (creatinine/eGFR).

SERUM ALDOSTERONE AND PLASMA RENIN

Order these tests as clinically indicated.

Aldosterone is a potent mineralocorticoid that regulates sodium, potassium, and water balance.

In combination, these tests distinguish between primary and secondary (more common) hyperaldosteronism.

TESTS FOR HYPOTHYROIDISM

Order these tests as clinically indicated:

- Start with TSH, which is the single best initial test for thyroid disorders.
- Follow up with a repeat TSH plus a T_4 if the initial TSH is elevated.

See: hypothyroidism, p. 37

URINE MICROSCOPY

Order this test as clinically indicated.

It may identify artifactual causes of pseudohyponatremia, including evidence of waxy casts (hypertriglyceridemia), and hyaline or granular casts
(paraproteinemia).

NEPHROLITHIASIS

KEYS TO WORKUP

The severe pain generated by renal colic primarily
comes from dilation, stretching, and spasm because of
acute ureteral obstruction. Often renal calculi can be
complicated by UTI and hematuria, which must be
distinguished by laboratory examination of the urine.

There are 4 principal types of renal calculi:

- calcium oxalate/phosphate stones, which can
  occur secondary to:
  - increased parathyroid hormone (PTH)
  - high calcium salt or protein intake
  - hyperoxaluria due to enteric overproduction
    or relative low calcium intake
  - factors that decrease stone solubility (e.g., low
    urine volumes, hypocitraturia, RTA type 1)
  - systemic causes (e.g., ethylene glycol
    ingestion or medullary sponge kidney)
  - high vitamin D intake

- struvite stones, which occur secondary to
  urinary tract infections
- cystine stones, due to chronic cystinuria
- uric acid stones (the only radiolucent stones)
  which are often due to:
  - excessive protein intake (gout)
  - chronic hyperuricosuria secondary to
    malignancy, ulcerative colitis, Crohn disease,
    or surgical jejunoileal bypass

LAB INVESTIGATIONS

24-HOUR URINE COLLECTION
Order this as an initial test.

Send any passed stones for analysis.

Note that this initial urine specimen will serve for follow-up tests, if it is refrigerated and if the tests are done within 2 to 4 days.

URINALYSIS
Order this as an initial test.

This test assesses bacterial nitrite (e.g., gram-negative bacteria), leukocyte esterase, protein, and specific gravity (see Table 7 for normal urinalysis values).

URINE CYSTINE AND URINE URIC ACID FROM 24-HOUR URINE COLLECTION
Order these as follow-up tests if the initial tests (or imaging) suggest stones.

These tests help determine:

- the type of stones
- whether the stones can be treated with radio-ablation

URINE MICROSCOPY
Depending on laboratory instrumentation, order this as a follow-up test if the results of urinalysis are abnormal, suggesting bacteriuria or hematuria (note that automated urinalysis analyzers will perform this automatically as part of routine urinalysis).

This test identifies cells, casts, and crystals.

URINE CULTURE AND ANTIBIOTIC SENSITIVITY
Order this as a follow-up test if you suspect UTI or if microscopy is positive.

POLYURIA

KEYS TO WORKUP

Polyuria has a wide range of possible underlying causes, which appropriate laboratory testing can distinguish:

- Screening urinalysis detects UTIs (the most common causes of polyuria).
- More specialized tests can determine the presence of osmotic and water dieresis related to endocrine dysfunction.

Polyuria is defined as more than 2 L to 3 L (2.1–3.2 qt) of urine production in a 24-hour period (see the breakdown that follows).

24-hour urine production*	Category
> 2 L	Polyuria
600 mL–2 L	Normal
100 mL–600 mL	Oliguria
< 100 mL	Anuria

*1 mL/min x 60 min/h x 24 h/d = 1.44 L/d

Polyuria is due to either:

- osmotic diuresis (urine osmolality > serum osmolality)
- water diuresis (urine osmolality < serum osmolality)

OSMOTIC DIURESIS

The causes of osmotic diuresis include:

- hyperglycemia (uncontrolled diabetes mellitus is a common cause of polyuria)
- mannitol or NaCl administration
- increased urea concentration (protein feeds, hypercatabolism due to burns and steroids, recovery from ARF)

WATER DIURESIS

Water deprivation testing can distinguish causes of water diuresis:

- If urine becomes hypertonic with water deprivation, the cause of polyuria is likely excessive intake (polydipsia).
- If urine remains hypotonic, the cause is likely excessive loss (DI).

Administration of desmopressin (e.g., DDAVP) can distinguish between:

- hypothalamic DI (urine osmolality increases by > 50% with desmopressin)
- nephrogenic DI (urine osmolality unchanged or increases < 50% with desmopressin)

LAB INVESTIGATIONS

URINALYSIS

Order this test as part of your initial workup (see Table 7 for normal urinalysis values).

URINE AND SERUM OSMOLALITY, AND URINE ELECTROLYTES

Order these tests as part of your initial workup (see Table 8 for normal urine electrolyte values).

Urine osmolality by random, timed, or 24-hour urine collection assesses:

- electrolyte and fluid balance
- the kidneys' ability to concentrate urine
- renal disease
- DI
- SIADH

Note that determination of both urine and serum osmolality aids in interpretation of results.

SERUM GLUCOSE

Order this test as part of your initial workup.

This test detects diabetes mellitus, a common cause of polyuria.

SERUM AND URINE ALDOSTERONE

Order these as follow-up tests if the initial tests show abnormal urine electrolytes.

Aldosterone is a potent mineralocorticoid that regulates sodium, potassium, and water balance.

ADH SUPPRESSION

Order this as a follow-up test if the initial tests show abnormal urine osmolality.

ADH controls the amount of water reabsorbed by the kidney:

- Inadequate ADH secretion results in DI.
- Excess ADH secretion (related to cancer—e.g., lung, pancreas, urinary tract, blood) results in SIADH.

URINARY FREQUENCY AND URGENCY, INCREASED

KEYS TO WORKUP

Laboratory tests are critical to distinguish many causes of increased urinary frequency and urgency.

Causes of increased urinary frequency can be either:

- extrinsic to the bladder:
  - vulvovaginitis or bladder compression (e.g., pregnancy)
  - systemic disorder (e.g., osmotic diuresis in diabetes)
  - stroke or neurologic disease affecting detrusor muscle function
  - diuretic medications
  - increased fluid intake

- intrinsic to the bladder:
  - small bladder volume
  - UTI (often with dysuria)
  - urinary obstruction secondary to BPH
  - prostate cancer
  - calculi

LAB INVESTIGATIONS

URINALYSIS
Begin with this test, to look for infection (see Table 7 for normal urinalysis values).

OTHER TESTS
Base decisions about other tests on the clinical situation.

Consider PSA in older males with BPH-like urinary obstructive symptoms to rule out carcinoma. Note other conditions, such as prostatitis, can also produce elevated PSA levels.

URINARY INCONTINENCE AND ENURESIS

KEYS TO WORKUP
Urinary incontinence, or involuntary leakage of urine, can happen for multiple reasons. Laboratory testing can help distinguish causes and identify those with underlying treatable medical conditions.

Urinary incontinence can be transient and easily reversible when due to any of the following:

- delirium, confusional states, or restricted mobility
- UTI
- atrophic urethritis or vaginitis
- pharmaceuticals
- psychological causes

- polyuria
- stool impaction or constipation

Urinary incontinence that is chronic and not easily reversed can be classified as follows:

- stress incontinence: from failure of urethral sphincter often after multiple pregnancies
- overflow incontinence: from impaired detrusor contraction due to neurologic deficits or bladder outlet obstruction
- urge incontinence: from detrusor overactivity

LAB INVESTIGATIONS

URINALYSIS

Order this as an initial test (see Table 7 for normal urinalysis values).

Urinalysis can identify:

- causes of polyuria (specific gravity, glucose, ketones)
- renal causes (protein, cells) contributing to urinary incontinence
- UTI (leukocyte esterase, nitrites)

OTHER TESTS

Select other tests depending on the clinical situation and the findings of the initial tests. These tests may include:

- tests for causes of excessive urine output (*see: polyuria, p. 117*)
- PSA levels: consider this in the case of older males with BPH-like urinary obstructive symptoms to rule out carcinoma (note that other conditions, such as prostatitis, can produce elevated PSA levels)
- urine cystine and uric acid levels: use this to assess patients with renal calculus formation and identify patients at risk for stone formation

- urine microscopy: this identifies cells, casts and crystals, and should be done whenever urinalysis is abnormal
- urine culture and antibiotic sensitivity: order this if microscopy is positive for UTI or if UTI is clinically suspected

FURTHER READING
Delaney MP, Price CP, Lamb EJ. Kidney disease. In: Burtis CA, Ashwood ER, Bruns DE, eds. 5th ed. *Tietz Textbook of Clinical Chemistry and Molecular Diagnostics.* St. Louis, MO: Saunders; 2012:1523–1608.

Gynecology and pregnancy

Dr. Christopher Naugler

ABBREVIATIONS

AFP	α_1-fetoprotein	MRI	magnetic resonance imaging
ALP	alkaline phosphatase	NT	nuchal translucency
ALT	alanine aminotransferase	PAPP-A	pregnancy-associated plasma protein A
AST	aspartate aminotransferase		
DHEA-S	dehydroepiandrosterone-sulfate	PCOS	polycystic ovary syndrome
E_2	estradiol	PT/INR	prothrombin time or international normalized ratio
E_3	estriol		
FSH	follicle-stimulating hormone	PTT	partial thromboplastin time
GBS	group B *Streptococcus*	T_3	triiodothyronine
GGT	γ-glutamyltransferase	T_4	thyroxine
hCG	human chorionic gonadotropin	TSH	thyroid-stimulating hormone (thyrotropin)
HIV	human immunodeficiency virus		
INR	international normalized ratio		
LH	luteinizing hormone		
MMR	measles-mumps-rubella vaccine		

DISORDERS AND CLINICAL PRESENTATIONS

GALACTORRHEA

KEYS TO WORKUP

The main differential diagnosis for galactorrhea is between:

- increased breast sensitivity to prolactin
- prolactin-producing pituitary tumour

LAB INVESTIGATIONS

PROLACTIN

An elevated prolactin level may indicate a pituitary tumour (prolactinoma). Other causes include certain medications, stress, hypothyroidism, and macroprolactinemia. Abnormal tests should be repeated.

PEARLS

Galactorrhea with persistently elevated prolactin levels is an indication for pituitary imaging (MRI).

HIRSUTISM, POLYCYSTIC OVARY SYNDROME

KEYS TO WORKUP

Polycystic ovary syndrome (PCOS) often comes to medical attention because of hirsutism secondary to hyperandrogenism. Laboratory testing aims to support or rule out a diagnosis of PCOS.

Despite the high prevalence of PCOS, the diagnosis and differential diagnosis remain confusing. This is in part due to the lack of a specific diagnostic test for the disorder.

LAB INVESTIGATIONS

See the breakdown that follows.[1]

Note that:

- All tests may not be necessary for all patients.
- Diagnosis is based on clinical-pathological correlation.

Lab test	Diagnostic objective
Dehydroepiandrosterone-sulfate (DHEA-S)	Adrenal tumour
24-hour urine free cortisol	Cushing syndrome *See: Cushing syndrome, p. 25*
Prolactin	Hyperprolactinemia
Total testosterone	Hyperthecosis Ovarian tumour
Thyroid-stimulating hormone (TSH)	Hypothyroidism *See: hypothyroidism, p. 37*
17-hydroxyprogesterone	Late-onset congenital adrenal hyperplasia
β-hCG	Pregnancy

IRREGULAR CYCLES IN YOUNGER WOMEN

KEYS TO WORKUP

Common causes of irregular cycles include:

- athletic training
- menarche
- menopause (*see: menopause, p. 129*)

For women who do not fit the common etiologies, the main considerations are:

- PCOS
- premature ovarian failure (patients < 40 years old)
- thyroid disease

History should help identify likely etiologies, and should guide decisions about laboratory tests.

LAB INVESTIGATIONS

TESTS FOR POLYCYSTIC OVARY SYNDROME
See: hirsutism, polycystic ovary syndrome, p. 124

TESTS FOR PREMATURE OVARIAN FAILURE

Order the following tests if you suspect premature ovarian failure:

- follicle-stimulating hormone (FSH)
- luteinizing hormone (LH)
- estradiol (E_2)

Premature ovarian failure is characterized by increased LH and FSH levels, and decreased E_2 levels.

TESTS FOR THYROID DISORDERS

Use the following tests to rule out thyroid disease (hyper- and hypothyroidism):

- TSH: start with this test, which is the single best initial test for thyroid disorders
- repeat TSH with T_4: follow up with these tests if the initial TSH is elevated, to confirm a diagnosis of hypothyroidism
- T_4: follow up with this test if the TSH is suppressed to confirm hyperthyroidism
- T_3: this is rarely indicated, and is useful only when TSH is suppressed but free T_4 is normal (a pattern known as T_3 toxicosis)

See: thyroid disorders, p. 33

PEARLS

FSH and LH should not be measured if the patient is taking oral contraceptives or medroxyprogesterone acetate (Provera).

MATERNAL SCREENING

KEYS TO SCREENING

Some prenatal tests are considered standard, and all pregnant women should receive these. Some regions also recommend other tests. Refer to local guidelines to ensure your patients receive all recommended tests.

LAB INVESTIGATIONS

FIRST PRENATAL VISIT

Standard tests include:

- blood type
- hepatitis B surface antigen
- HIV antibody
- red cell antibody screen
- Rubella antibody titres
- syphilis serology
- urine culture
  - Note that asymptomatic bacteriuria is generally not treated, except in pregnant women where the asymptomatic presence of more than 100 000 colony-forming units per mL of urine increase the chances of acute pyelonephritis.
- oral glucose tolerance test, for women at high risk of diabetes (family history of diabetes, obesity, prior gestational diabetes)
  - Protocols for oral glucose tolerance tests vary, but generally include a 50 g screening test followed by a 75 g or 100 g confirmatory test for those with positive screens.
  - Note that the cut-off for a positive oral glucose tolerance test is different for pregnant women and nonpregnant women.
- varicella antibody (if immunity is not known)

28 WEEKS GESTATION

Order an oral glucose tolerance test (standard at 28 weeks).

35 TO 37 WEEKS GESTATION

Order vaginal and rectal cultures for group B *Streptococcus* (GBS) (standard at 35 to 37 weeks).

PEARLS

Ideally, women should get tested for rubella antibody prior to pregnancy, as the MMR vaccine is contraindicated during pregnancy.

GBS is the most common cause of life-threatening infection in newborns. Antibiotic treatment of the mother decreases GBS infections by 20 fold.

MATERNAL SERUM PRENATAL SCREEN (FETAL PRENATAL TESTING)

All provinces and territories have prenatal screening programs. The information presented here is meant as an overview only.

KEYS TO SCREENING

All pregnant women should receive fetal prenatal screening regardless of maternal age or family history.

There are 2 main options for fetal testing (the choice of test depends on local availability and practice guidelines):

- first trimester screen
- second trimester screen

These screening tests are not diagnostic, but can indicate a higher risk for conditions such as Down syndrome, trisomy 18, trisomy 13, and neural tube defects.

Women with higher risk ("positive") screens may be offered additional testing such as amniocentesis and counselling.

LAB INVESTIGATIONS

FIRST TRIMESTER SCREEN

This screen is generally done between:

- 8 and 13 6/7 weeks gestation

It consists of:

- blood tests for pregnancy-associated plasma protein A (PAPP-A) and human chorionic gonadotropin (β-hCG)
- ultrasound for fetal nuchal translucency (NT)

SECOND TRIMESTER SCREEN

This screen is generally done between:

- 15 3/7 to 16 3/7 weeks gestation

It consists of 4 blood tests:

- α_1-fetoprotein (AFP)
- estriol (E_3)
- β-hCG
- inhibin

PEARLS

Make sure to accurately convey gestational age to the laboratory: an incorrect gestational age may result in false-positive or false-negative results. For this reason, dates are generally confirmed by ultrasound.

MENOPAUSE

KEYS TO WORKUP

You can generally diagnose menopause on the basis of history. Laboratory confirmation is not necessary in the majority of cases.

LAB INVESTIGATIONS

Tests to confirm menopause (not generally recommended) include:

- estradiol (E_2)
- FSH
- LH

During menopause, E_2 levels fall, and LH and FSH levels increase.

PAPANICOLAOU (PAP) TEST
See: routine screening, p. 243

VAGINAL BLEEDING, ABNORMAL

KEYS TO WORKUP
In premenopausal women, abnormal vaginal bleeding has a specific cause in slightly over half of cases.

The following are key to diagnosis:

- clinical examination of the vagina and cervix
- laboratory testing
- ultrasound of the uterus

LAB INVESTIGATIONS

INITIAL TESTS
All women with abnormal vaginal bleeding should have the following tests:

- CBC, INR, PTT, TSH (order as a panel)
- endometrial biopsy
- Pap test

Premenopausal women should also have (prior to endometrial biopsy):

- a pregnancy test (urine qualitative β-hCG or serum quantitative β-hCG)

If the results of these tests and uterine imaging (e.g., transvaginal ultrasound) are normal, consider a diagnosis of dysfunctional uterine bleeding.

OTHER TESTS
Depending on the presence of other symptoms, also consider and test for less common causes including:

- Cushing disease: measure cortisol (*see: Cushing disease, p. 26*)

- hepatic disease: measure ALP, ALT, GGT (and, as indicated, AST, direct and indirect bilirubin, PT/INR)
- prolactinoma: measure prolactin

PEARLS

Postmenopausal bleeding (defined as any vaginal bleeding 1 year after menstruation has stopped) is always abnormal and requires evaluation.

REFERENCES

1   Sheehan MT. Polycystic ovarian syndrome: diagnosis and management. *Clin Med Res*. 2004;2(1):13–27. http://dx.doi.org/10.3121/cmr.2.1.13. Medline:15931331

FURTHER READING

Cunniff C; American Academy of Pediatrics Committee on Genetics. Prenatal screening and diagnosis for pediatricians. *Pediatrics*. 2004;114(3):889–894. http://dx.doi.org/10.1542/peds.2004-1368. Medline:15342871

Telner DE, Jakubovicz D. Approach to diagnosis and management of abnormal uterine bleeding. *Can Fam Physician*. 2007;53(1):58–64. Medline:17872610

Hematology

Dr. Launny Faulkner

ABBREVIATIONS

ALP	alkaline phosphatase	GI	gastrointestinal
ALT	alanine aminotransferase	Hb	hemoglobin
ANA	antinuclear antibody	HBV	hepatitis B virus
aPTT	activated partial thromboplastin time	Hct	hematocrit
		HELLP	**h**emolysis, **el**evated liver enzymes, **l**ow **p**latelet count
ASA	acetylsalicylic acid		
AST	aspartate aminotransferase	HIT	heparin-induced thrombocytopenia
AT	antithrombin		
CBC	complete blood count	HIV	human immunodeficiency virus
CHF	congestive heart failure	HSV	herpes simplex virus
CMV	cytomegalovirus	HUS	hemolytic uremic syndrome
BUN	blood urea nitrogen	ITP	immune thrombocytopenia
DAT	direct antiglobulin test	IVC	inferior vena cava
DIC	disseminated intravascular coagulation	LDH	lactate dehydrogenase
		LFT	liver function test
DVT	deep vein thrombosis	MAHA	microangiopathic hemolytic anemia
EBV	Epstein-Barr virus		
EDTA	ethylenediaminetetraacetic acid	MCH	mean corpuscular hemoglobin
EPO	erythropoietin	MCHC	mean corpuscular hemoglobin concentration
FNA	fine needle aspiration		
G6PD	glucose-6-phosphate dehydrogenase deficiency	MCV	mean corpuscular volume
		OCP	oral contraceptive
GGT	γ-glutamyltransferase	PE	pulmonary embolism

PSA	prostate-specific antigen	TB	tuberculosis
PT/INR	prothrombin time or international normalized ratio	TIBC	total iron binding capacity
		TTP	thrombotic thrombocytopenic purpura
RBC	red blood cell		
RDW	red blood cell distribution width	TSH	thyroid-stimulating hormone (thyrotropin)
RF	rheumatoid factor		
SLE	systemic lupus erythematosus	VTE	venous thromboembolism
SPE	serum protein electrophoresis	vWF	von Willebrand factor
STD	sexually transmitted disease	WBC	white blood cell

DISORDERS AND CLINICAL PRESENTATIONS

Anemia

The initial workup of many clinical presentations calls for a CBC, which may reveal a low hemoglobin level. Whether or not symptoms of anemia are present, low hemoglobin may be the first sign of significant underlying disease and warrants further investigation.

Two common approaches to anemia are to divide diagnoses mechanistically (see Table 9) or morphologically (see Table 10). Along with the clinical history, information from a peripheral smear may help guide the next steps in testing.

Table 9. Classification of anemia by mechanism

Decreased production	Increased destruction	Blood loss
Iron deficiency	**Congenital**	**Obvious**
Vitamin B$_{12}$ or folate deficiency	Hemoglobinopathies (e.g., sickle cell disease)	Hematemesis
Anemia of chronic disease	RBC membrane disorders (e.g., hereditary spherocytosis)	Melena
Aplastic anemia		Menometrorrhagia
Myelodysplasia	RBC metabolism disorders (e.g., G6PD deficiency)	Trauma
Marrow infiltration	Thalassemia	

Continued on p. 135

Continued from p. 134

Decreased production	Increased destruction	Blood loss
Marrow suppression (drugs, radiation, infection) Decreased hormonal stimulation (e.g., low EPO in renal failure, hypothyroidism, hypogonadism)	**Acquired**	**Occult**
	Immune Nonimmune (e.g., malaria)	GI bleed (e.g., ulcer, malignancy) Menorrhagia
		Induced
		Blood donation Excessive blood draws Hemodialysis losses

Table 10. Classification of anemia by morphology

Low MCV	Normal MCV	High MCV
Anemia of chronic disease (e.g., renal, liver, endocrinopathy, chronic inflammation/infection)	Acute bleed	Alcohol
Copper deficiency	Anemia of chronic disease (e.g., renal, liver, endocrinopathy, chronic inflammatory/infection)	Vitamin B_{12} or folate deficiency
Disorders of iron metabolism		Drugs
Hemoglobinopathies	Hemolysis	Hypothyroidism
Iron deficiency	Marrow infiltration	Liver disease
Lead poisoning	Marrow suppression	Myelodysplasia
Thalassemia		Reticulocytosis

SOURCES OF ERROR

As always, keep sources of error in the differential for any abnormal test result.

In particular, the following may interfere with test accuracy:

- under- or overfilling collection tubes
- allowing samples to sit too long at room temperature
- increased turbidity due to hyperlipidemia

Be wary of discrepant or unexpected results, remembering that errors in the measured values

(Hb, RBC count, MCV) will also affect the values derived from them (Hct, MCH, MCHC).

ANEMIA WITH LOW MCV

KEYS TO WORKUP

Microcytic anemia is characteristic of decreased or defective hemoglobin synthesis, and is often accompanied by a low mean corpuscular hemoglobin concentration (MCHC) (see the breakdown that follows). Iron deficiency is by far the most likely diagnosis in both adults and children, followed by thalassemia and chronic inflammation.

Reduced iron availability	Reduced heme synthesis	Reduced functional globin production
Severe iron deficiency	Lead poisoning	Hemoglobinopathies
Chronic inflammation	Sideroblastic anemia	Thalassemic states
Copper deficiency		
Disorders of iron metabolism (rare)		

LAB INVESTIGATIONS

See Figure 6.

Initial CBC results may help distinguish iron deficiency and thalassemia:

- Elevated platelets and a high red blood cell distribution width (RDW) favour iron deficiency.
- Normal RDW with a high RBC count favours thalassemia.

A ferritin is the single most sensitive and specific test for iron deficiency in the outpatient setting:

- Low levels reflect severely depleted iron stores.

- Elevated ferritin may represent an inability to mobilize iron stores for use in heme synthesis, and is seen in conditions causing acute or chronic inflammation (anemia of chronic disease).

If ferritin is inconclusive, as may be seen in early or partially treated iron deficiency, a peripheral blood smear may still reveal characteristic findings (e.g., elliptocytes or "pencil cells").

Ancillary tests such as total iron binding capacity (TIBC), transferrin saturation, and iron concentration lack specificity and are of limited diagnostic value in most patients. Current guidelines discourage their use, instead recommending a trial of iron therapy. In the absence of malabsorption, reticulocytosis should be present within 7 days of initiating therapy, with an increase in hemoglobin of 10–20 g/L (1–2 g/dL) within 2 to 4 weeks.

Order a peripheral smear whenever the diagnosis remains unclear or red cell indices suggest a disease process other than poor availability of iron. Based on patient history and morphologic findings, a pathologist may make a diagnosis or recommend further testing, such as hemoglobin electrophoresis or bone marrow biopsy.

SOURCES OF ERROR
If present, large platelets may be counted as small red cells and falsely skew the mean corpuscular volume (MCV) toward microcytosis.

PEARLS
Ferritin is an acute phase reactant, and may be elevated in acutely ill patients or in the presence of inflammation.

When diagnosing iron deficiency, it is imperative to find the root cause (see Table 11). Unless specific dietary restrictions are present, inadequate intake is uncommon in North America.

Table 11. Causes of iron deficiency anemia

Process	Specific etiology
Inadequate dietary intake	Alcoholism, poorly balanced vegetarian diet, "tea and toast" diet
Insufficient intake to meet increased requirements	Normal childhood growth, menstruation, pregnancy and delivery, lactation
Decreased absorption	Chronic renal failure, gastric/duodenal pathology (celiac disease, Crohn disease, chronic gastritis, gastric bypass), medications that bind iron, high intake of foods that inhibit iron binding (dairy, coffee and tea, high-fibre foods, carbonated drinks)
Increased blood loss	Hemolysis, menorrhagia, GI bleeding, intestinal parasites, hematuria, surgery, trauma, frequent blood donation

ANEMIA WITH NORMAL MCV

KEYS TO WORKUP

This large and heterogeneous category can be divided mechanistically by the presence or absence of reticulocytosis:

- A normal or decreased reticulocyte count signals decreased production.
- An elevated count signals increased destruction or loss.

The number of white cells and platelets may point toward a certain etiology, and a peripheral smear is especially valuable in the workup of normocytic anemia.

LAB INVESTIGATIONS

See Figure 7.

If reticulocytosis is normal or decreased, early iron deficiency, or chronic disease or inflammation, are most likely. Appropriate tests include:

LAB LITERACY FOR CANADIAN DOCTORS **139**

- ferritin
- tests for specific entities (e.g., hypothyroidism, renal failure) as guided by the clinical assessment

A sustained increase in WBCs or platelets suggests myelodysplasia or hematologic malignancy, while a decrease suggests marrow suppression or replacement.

If the cause of anemia is not apparent or the evidence suggests marrow failure or infiltration, request a peripheral smear and consider a bone marrow biopsy.

An increase in reticulocytes confirms an appropriate marrow response to RBC loss or destruction. Acute blood loss, hemolysis, and hypersplenism top the differential.

See: splenomegaly, p. 155

TESTS FOR HEMOLYSIS

An increased lactate dehydrogenase (LDH) with a reduction in haptoglobin confirms hemolysis (over 90% specific in combination). Elevated unconjugated bilirubin also supports this diagnosis.

A peripheral smear is paramount in the evaluation of hemolysis; both congenital and acquired diagnoses display characteristic changes in red cell morphology.

A direct antiglobulin test is both sensitive and specific to confirm immune-mediated hemolysis.

PEARLS

Hemolysis or blood loss can be associated with a low reticulocyte count if there is a concurrent disorder that impairs RBC production (e.g., iron deficiency, infection, recent chemotherapy).

ANEMIA WITH HIGH MCV

KEYS TO WORKUP

The most common causes of macrocytic anemia are drugs (including alcohol), liver disease, and vitamin B_{12} deficiency. Folate deficiency is exceedingly rare in North America. Brisk reticulocytosis may elevate the MCV, but is not considered true macrocytosis, as mature red cells are normal in size.

LAB INVESTIGATIONS

See Figure 8.

A peripheral smear may provide clues to the specific abnormality present.

Macrocytosis may be the only abnormality in drug effects, though medications that interfere with nucleic acid synthesis (e.g., methotrexate, chemo-therapeutics) may create a megaloblastic picture similar to vitamin B_{12} or folic acid deficiency. An MCV over 115 fL, oval macrocytes, and hypersegmented neutrophils are classic megaloblastic findings, though hypersegmentation may also be seen in iron deficiency.

Though less specific, features suggestive of liver disease (e.g., target cells) warrant liver function testing in otherwise asymptomatic patients. Such tests may include ALP, ALT, AST, direct and indirect bilirubin, GGT, and PT/INR.

Screening for hypothyroidism in the absence of other symptoms remains controversial, but may be justified in the appropriate clinical setting.

SOURCES OF ERROR

Excessively high values for MCV may be measured when cold agglutinins are present, causing clumps of RBCs to be counted as single cells. Warming the specimen (and reagents) to body temperature prior to a repeat count should return the MCV to normal, and confirm the presence of a cold agglutinin.

Hyperosmolar states, such as uncontrolled diabetes mellitus or dehydration, may also result in falsely elevated MCV. Red cells that have adjusted to the higher osmolarity will swell when placed in (comparatively) hypo-osmolar testing reagents.

PEARLS

On occasion, elevated plasma proteins may cause red cells to stack together and falsely increase the measured MCV. Rouleaux formation on peripheral smear is indicative of such an occurrence, and though not a true macrocytic anemia requires further investigation due to its association with inflammatory states and multiple myeloma. A serum protein electrophoresis (SPE) will differentiate a monoclonal population from the elevation seen in inflammatory states.

Bleeding and bruising

The hemostatic process involves a complex interplay among:

- platelet number and function
- vascular integrity
- coagulation factors
- fibrinolysis

Disorders of hemostasis manifest as bleeding that is spontaneous, excessive, or delayed in onset.

A thorough bleeding history should guide initial testing based on the suspected mechanism:

- disorders of primary hemostasis: abnormal function of platelets or vessels, causing mucosal or minor cutaneous bleeding
- disorders of secondary hemostasis: defects in coagulation, causing severe or delayed bleeding into deep tissues and joints

DISORDERS OF PLATELETS

KEYS TO WORKUP

QUANTITATIVE DEFECTS

Thrombocytopenia alone does not usually lead to spontaneous or excessive bleeding unless the platelet count falls below $30 \times 10^9/L$ ($30 \times 10^3/\mu L$).

The differential diagnosis of quantitative defects is divided by mechanism (see Table 12).

Table 12. Differential diagnosis of quantitative defects of platelets

Mechanism	Etiologies
Decreased production	Marrow suppression • viral infection • chemotherapy or radiation • alcohol toxicity • HIV (direct megakaryocyte inhibition) Congenital aplasia or hypoplasia Vitamin B_{12} or folic acid deficiency
Increased destruction	Drugs (e.g., quinine, valproic acid) Infection (mononucleosis, CMV, HIV) Immune-mediated conditions: • immune thrombocytopenia (ITP) • SLE • heparin-induced thrombocytopenia (HIT) • antiphospholipid syndrome • alloimmune response (post transfusion or transplant) MAHAs: • disseminated intravascular coagulation (DIC) • thrombotic thrombocytopenic purpura (TTP) • hemolytic uremic syndrome (HUS) • HELLP syndrome Physical destruction: • cardiopulmonary bypass • giant cavernous hemangiomata • large aortic aneurysm • intravascular metastasis

Continued on p. 143

Continued from p. 142

Mechanism	Etiologies
Sequestration	Normal state: • 1/3 of circulating platelets sequestered in the spleen Portal hypertension with congestive splenomegaly: • up to 90% of circulating platelets sequestered in the spleen, but available platelet mass unchanged (unlikely to present as bleeding)

FUNCTIONAL DEFECTS

Defects of platelet function include:

- acquired defects due to drugs (e.g., ASA) or metabolic disease (e.g., renal failure)
- congenital defects (rare)

DYSFUNCTION OF VON WILLEBRAND FACTOR

Due to its intimate role in platelet adherence, dysfunction of von Willebrand factor (vWF) also presents as mucocutaneous bleeding.

It is the most common inherited bleeding disorder, but rare acquired forms have also been described.

LAB INVESTIGATIONS

See Figure 9.

A CBC is the first test to order for any bleeding patient. If platelets are low, request a peripheral smear to exclude pseudothrombocytopenia, which may be caused by in vitro agglutination of platelets in the presence of ethylenediaminetetraacetic acid (EDTA). Though uncommon, this phenomenon can be avoided in susceptible patients by using alternative anticoagulants for sample collection, such as heparin or sodium citrate. Clinical history should guide further investigation as to the cause of a true thrombocytopenia.

Patients with von Willebrand disease may have a prolonged aPTT due to a mild deficiency of factor VIII (normally stabilized by vWF). Specific diagnostic tests include:

- quantitative immunoassays for vWF antigen
- functional assays such as ristocetin cofactor activity

Repeat testing may be required to establish the diagnosis as factor levels can vary over time: vWF may be elevated in pregnancy, oral contraceptive use, or liver disease.

Most tests of platelet function measure agglutination in response to various additives:

- If a patient experiences mucosal bleeding while on medication which may interfere with platelet function, consider a trial of an alternative medication before pursuing functional lab testing.
- If, however, bleeding persists and more likely causes have been excluded, contact your local laboratory to determine which tests of platelet function are available.

DISORDERS OF VASCULATURE

KEYS TO WORKUP

Vessel wall integrity may be impaired by:

- older age
- medications (classically steroids)
- vasculitides
- connective tissue disorders
- primary vessel abnormalities (e.g., hereditary telangiectasia)

Suspect a primary vessel defect when investigations for platelets and coagulation have been normal. The diagnosis is primarily clinical, but consider referral for genetic testing if a specific disorder is suspected (e.g., Ehlers-Danlos).

LAB INVESTIGATIONS
See Figure 9.

See: disorders of coagulation (next), and disorders of platelets, p. 142

DISORDERS OF COAGULATION

KEYS TO WORKUP
Coagulopathies are more commonly acquired than congenital.

The following may present as clotting-factor deficiencies:

- iatrogenic anticoagulation
- inhibitors (drugs or autoantibodies)
- liver disease
- vitamin K deficiency

Deficiencies may also arise from increased consumption of clotting factors—for example, from major trauma or DIC. These are usually apparent from the clinical setting, but may be confirmed with laboratory testing.

LAB INVESTIGATIONS
See Figure 10.

PT/INR AND aPTT
The 2 staple tests of coagulation are:

- activated partial thromboplastin time (aPTT)
- prothrombin time (PT/INR)

PROLONGED PT/INR
This signals a defect in the extrinsic pathway, commonly due to deficiency in vitamin K (fat malabsorption, antibiotic use, poor nutrition) or warfarin therapy.

PROLONGED aPTT

This suggests a problem with the intrinsic pathway.

Causes include:

- congenital factor deficiencies
- autoantibodies against coagulation factors
- drug effects (e.g., heparin)

Patients with von Willebrand disease may have a prolonged aPTT due to a mild deficiency of factor VIII (normally stabilized by vWF).

Also note that:

- Some factor deficiencies prolong aPTT in the absence of any bleeding tendency.
- Certain autoantibodies (e.g., the lupus anticoagulant) may in fact promote coagulation despite a prolonged aPTT in vitro.

PROLONGED PT/INR AND aPTT

This suggests a deficiency, defect, or inhibition of a factor in the common pathway.

Possible causes include:

- concomitant administration of both heparin and warfarin
- heparin overdose: though the effects of heparin are best monitored with aPTT, it will also prolong PT/INR in supratherapeutic doses
- Warfarin overdose, severe vitamin K deficiency, and significant liver disease: although PT/INR is more sensitive to low levels of vitamin K–dependent factors, severe depletion also prolongs aPTT
- DIC: may prolong 1 or both of the PT/INR and aPTT, and is accompanied by a low platelet count on CBC; the diagnosis is confirmed by an elevated D-dimer, decreased plasma fibrinogen, and schistocytes on peripheral smear (see Figure 10c)

FURTHER INVESTIGATION FOR SUSPECTED FACTOR DEFICIENCIES OR INHIBITORS

Mixing studies (see Figure 10b) distinguish between prolonged coagulation caused by:

- deficiency (or absence) of a factor (corrects on mixing)
- presence of a coagulation-factor inhibitor (does not correct or only partially corrects on mixing)

Specific assays will be performed as per laboratory protocol for identification. Immunologic assays can also measure factor levels, but do not detect a functionally abnormal factor that is present at normal levels. Factor inhibitors (such as autoantibodies or interfering substances such as heparin) have been described in association with malignancy, lymphoproliferative disorders, pregnancy, and rheumatologic disease, and thus may warrant further investigation.

Lupus anticoagulants (e.g., antiphospholipid antibodies) may also prolong the aPTT without correction on mixing. Paradoxically, this syndrome is usually associated with a tendency toward thrombosis rather than bleeding.

SOURCES OF ERROR

Remember to keep sources of error in the differential for any lab result:

- Under- or overfilling collection tubes will result in an incorrect ratio of plasma to anticoagulant, artificially prolonging or shortening the clotting time respectively.
- Drawing blood into an incorrect tube (e.g., EDTA, heparin) or through a heparinized line will falsely elevate PTT, while increased turbidity (e.g., hyperlipidemia, very high WBC) will shorten them.

- Samples must be sent to the lab within 2 hours if kept at room temperature, and within 4 hours if refrigerated, to ensure accurate results.

Other hematologic disorders

THROMBOSIS AND THROMBOPHILIA

KEYS TO WORKUP

Most patients with an established thrombotic event have 1 or more acquired or congenital risk factors (see Table 13).

If there is no readily apparent cause, begin by investigating for conditions such as pregnancy, occult malignancy, or inflammatory bowel disease as guided by the clinical history.

Screening for inherited thrombophilia is controversial: evidence suggests it does not change management or improve outcomes. However, most sources agree that in patients with unexplained or recurrent deep vein thrombosis (DVT) or pulmonary embolism (PE), or a strong family history of venous thromboembolism, testing for the most common forms of inherited thrombophilia is appropriate. These include the factor V Leiden mutation and the prothrombin gene mutation, together accounting for 60% of cases.

Table 13. Risk factors for deep vein thrombosis and pulmonary embolism

Acquired	Congenital
Physical:	Inherited:
• recent major surgery	• factor V Leiden mutation
• central venous catheter present	• prothrombin gene mutation
• trauma	• protein S deficiency
• immobilization	• protein C deficiency
• prior thrombotic event	• antithrombin (AT) deficiency
• thoracic outlet compression	• dysfibrinogenemia (rare)

Continued on p. 149

Continued from p. 148

Acquired	Congenital
Hormonal: • pregnancy • oral contraceptive use • hormone replacement therapy • tamoxifen, thalidomide, lenalidomide therapy Drug related: • heparin therapy Medical conditions: • myeloproliferative disorders (polycythemia vera, essential thrombocythemia) • antiphospholipid syndrome • malignancy • congestive heart failure • nephrotic syndrome • inflammatory bowel disease • paroxysmal nocturnal hemoglobinuria	Noninherited: • congenital malformations of the inferior vena cava (IVC)

LAB INVESTIGATIONS

See Figure 11.

Clinical assessment should guide initial laboratory investigations of patients with venous thromboembolism (VTE). Initial tests may include:

- CBC
- chemistry panel: BUN, creatinine, electrolytes, glucose
- liver function tests: ALP, ALT, GGT (and, as indicated, AST, direct and indirect bilirubin, PT/INR)
- urinalysis
- prostate-specific antigen (PSA) measurement (consider for men older than 50)

An elevated hemoglobin or platelet count may represent a myeloproliferative disorder, or may be secondary to an occult neoplasm. Low platelets while on heparin should prompt consideration of heparin-induced thrombocytopenia and thrombosis. A peripheral smear will give further direction, and may also reveal signs of chronic DIC.

The primary utility of coagulation tests is to detect factor deficiencies or inhibitors that prolong clotting times. A shortened PT/INR or aPTT usually reflects poor sample collection or preparation. In rare cases, it may signal increased factor activity in vivo, as seen in malignancy or chronic DIC (particularly, a shortened aPTT).

A prolonged aPTT that does not correct on 1:1 mixing with normal plasma (mixing study) suggests antiphospholipid antibody syndrome, which predisposes to thrombosis in vivo despite its anticoagulant effect in vitro. Additional specialized clotting assays (e.g., Russell viper venom time) facilitate the diagnosis.

For a patient with suspected inherited thrombophilia, a number of laboratory and genetic tests are available:

- Factor V Leiden: because of interference with other assays, factor V Leiden must be ruled out before proceeding with other testing. The most cost-effective test for factor V Leiden is an aPTT-based functional clotting assay, which is both sensitive and specific. Patients may be genotyped for the mutation, but this is not necessary.
- Protein C or S deficiency: functional assays provide the best way to screen for deficiency of protein C or S; antigenic testing detects quantitative but not qualitative defects.

- Antithrombin deficiency: functional assays also diagnose antithrombin deficiency; all currently recognized subtypes are detected making this the single best screening test for the disorder.
- There is no reliable functional assay for mutant prothrombin, which must be detected by genetic analysis.

SOURCES OF ERROR

The influence of acute thrombosis, comorbid illness, or anticoagulant therapy on plasma protein concentrations can lead to incorrect diagnoses.

Wait at least 2 weeks after the completion of anticoagulant therapy before proceeding with functional testing. If it is unsafe to discontinue anticoagulation, testing first-degree relatives may confirm a hereditary thrombophilia. Alternatively, investigation may be undertaken by changing to an anticoagulant that does not interfere with the testing method (e.g., protein C or S deficiency may be detected while on heparin but not warfarin).

LYMPHADENOPATHY

KEYS TO WORKUP

The cause of lymphadenopathy is often clear from history and physical exam.

In more difficult cases, diagnosis may require laboratory tests and lymph node biopsy. Along with clinical assessment, testing may be guided by whether the lymphadenopathy is generalized or localized (see Tables 14, 15, and 16).

Table 14. Causes of regional lymphadenopathy

Region	Causes
Cervical	Infection • local bacterial or viral • systemic infections (EBV, CMV, toxoplasmosis) • tuberculosis Lymphoma Kikuchi disease Metastatic carcinoma (especially metastatic oropharyngeal squamous cell carcinoma)
Supraclavicular	Malignancy • lung • esophagus • mediastinum • GI • kidneys • prostate • ovaries/testes Infection
Axillary	Infection (e.g., cat scratch disease) Malignancy • breast • other Breast implants
Epitrochlear	Infection • forearm or hand • secondary syphilis • tularemia Lymphoma Sarcoidosis
Inguinal	Infection • lower extremity • sexually transmitted Malignancy • skin of lower extremities • cervix • vulva • skin of trunk • rectum/anus • ovary • penis

Table 15. Causes of generalized lymphadenopathy

Common	Uncommon
Infectious mononucleosis	Castleman disease
Mycobacterial infection	Kikuchi disease
SLE	Angioimmunoblastic T-cell lymphoma
Medications	Inflammatory pseudotumour
HIV infection	Amyloidosis

Table 16. Causes of peripheral lymphadenopathy

Process	Specific etiology
Infectious	**Bacterial:** cellulitis, streptococcal pharyngitis, cat scratch disease, tularemia, yersinia, diphtheria, chancroid, brucellosis, leptospirosis, typhoid
	Viral: HIV, EBV, CMV, HSV, HBV, measles, mumps, rubella
	Mycobacterial: TB, atypical mycobacteria
	Fungal: *Cryptococcus*, Coccidia, *Histoplasma*
	Protozoal: toxoplasma, *Leishmania*
	Spirochetal: secondary syphilis, Lyme disease
Neoplastic	Lymphoproliferative neoplasm, leukemia/lymphoma, metastatic carcinoma
Immune/autoimmune	Serum sickness, drug reaction, Kikuchi disease, Kawasaki disease, SLE, rheumatoid arthritis, dermatomyositis, histiocytosis
Endocrine	Hypothyroidism, Addison disease
Other	Sarcoidosis, amyloidosis, lipid storage diseases, Castleman disease, inflammatory pseudotumour, Still disease, Churg-Strauss syndrome

LAB INVESTIGATIONS
See Figure 12.

TESTS FOR GENERALIZED LYMPHADENOPATHY
Patients with generalized lymphadenopathy without apparent cause should have the following:

- CBC
- WBC differential

- possibly a chest X-ray (consult imaging guidelines for further recommendations in the workup of adenopathy)

Other tests to consider include:

- peripheral smear: may reveal signs of infection or other systemic disease
- heterophile antibody test (mono test), TB skin test, antinuclear antibodies (ANA), and tests for syphilis or HIV: typically have low yield without a more specific indication, but should be ordered before proceeding to biopsy if enlarged nodes do not resolve

TESTS FOR LOCALIZED LYMPHADENOPATHY

When there is no clear diagnosis for localized lymphadenopathy and no evidence of infection on CBC, patients can be observed for 3 to 4 weeks as long as there is no suggestion of malignancy. If symptoms do not resolve or declare themselves during this time, obtain a biopsy specimen of the most abnormal node.

Biopsy options include:

- open biopsy: allows evaluation of architecture, microorganisms, and abnormal cell populations; always the best choice when an intact node is accessible
- core needle biopsy: provides tissue for special testing and preserves some architectural information; a reasonable alternative to open biopsy when an intact node is not easily accessible
- fine needle aspiration for cytology: has a significant false-negative rate due to sampling error and lack of architecture; can be useful in combination with core needle biopsy, when searching for recurrence of cancer, or in centres where open biopsy is not available

Notify the pathologist in advance that you are performing a lymph node biopsy and send the tissue in the fresh state (i.e., unfixed). If clinical suspicion remains after a negative biopsy, a second attempt (preferably open biopsy) should be performed.

SPLENOMEGALY

KEYS TO WORKUP

The differential diagnosis for splenomegaly has significant overlap with that of lymphadenopathy (see Table 17). Even when presenting in isolation, the initial workup remains quite similar. Imaging (not covered in this guide) may also play an important role in the diagnosis.

Table 17. Causes of splenomegaly

Process	Specific etiology
Congestive	Cirrhosis
	Heart failure
	Thrombosis of portal, hepatic, or splenic veins
Malignant	Hematologic (lymphoma, leukemia, polycythemia vera, multiple myeloma, essential thrombocythemia)
	Metastatic solid tumours
	Primary splenic tumours
Infection	Viral: hepatitis, infectious mononucleosis, cytomegalovirus
	Bacterial: *Salmonella*, *Brucella*, tuberculosis
	Parasitic: malaria, schistosomiasis, toxoplasmosis, leishmaniasis
	Infective endocarditis
	Fungal

Continued on p. 156

Continued from p. 155

Process	Specific etiology
Inflammation	Sarcoidosis
	Serum sickness
	SLE
	Rheumatoid arthritis (Felty syndrome)
Infiltrative	Gaucher disease
	Niemann-Pick disease
	Amyloidosis
	Glycogen storage disease
	Langerhans cell histiocytosis
	Hemophagocytic lymphohistiocytosis
	Rosai-Dorfman disease
Hypersplenic states	Acute or chronic hemolytic anemia
	Sickle cell disease
	Following use of granulocyte colony-stimulating factor

LAB INVESTIGATIONS
See Figure 13.

Order the following tests as an initial panel:

- CBC
- WBC differential
- peripheral smear
- liver function tests: ALP, ALT, GGT (and, as indicated, AST, direct and indirect bilirubin, PT/INR)

A blood smear may reveal signs of infection—occasionally even specific organisms—as well as myeloproliferative disorders, hematologic malignancy, hemolytic anemia, or hypersplenism.

Splenic biopsy is rarely performed and usually unnecessary; a liver or bone marrow biopsy is more likely to yield the diagnosis.

WHITE BLOOD COUNT, ELEVATED

KEYS TO WORKUP

Clinicians often encounter abnormalities in either the absolute white blood count and/or the white cell differential, often as incidental findings on complete blood counts ordered to assess anemia.

Table 18 shows the most common causes of increased and decreased numbers of white cells. Remember that infants and children normally have higher lymphocyte counts. A mildly elevated white cell count raises the question of a reactive leukocytosis versus a more sinister etiology. Mild deviations from normal in the absence of other worrisome symptoms can generally be retested with a follow-up CBC in 4 weeks to ensure resolution.

Considerable confusion exists as to when to further investigate lymphocytosis. Most cases are due to transient viral illness; however, a small proportion of patients have an underlying lymphoproliferative disorder or a developing leukemia. In general,

Table 18. Common causes of white blood cell count abnormalities

Cell	Causes of increased counts	Causes of decreased counts
Neutrophils	Infection, exercise, pregnancy, steroids	Infection, drug reaction, autoimmune disorder
Lymphocytes	Viral infection, drug reaction, lymphoproliferative disorder	Viral infection, drug reaction
Monocytes	Chronic infection, inflammation, myelodysplastic syndrome	N/A
Eosinophils	Allergy, asthma, parasitic infection, other systemic disease	N/A
Basophils	Allergy, viral infection, myelodysplastic syndrome, drug reaction	N/A

acute leukemias present with a markedly elevated lymphocyte count and may show concomitant thrombocytopenia and anemia. However, some leukemias may present with much lower than expected white cell counts.

LAB INVESTIGATIONS

CBC

For any mild deviation in white cell counts that is asymptomatic, start by ordering a repeat CBC in 4 to 6 weeks to assess for resolution.

PERIPHERAL BLOOD SMEAR

For significant abnormalities or deviations that persist over time, the first test to order is the microscopic evaluation of a peripheral blood smear.

OTHER TESTS

The evaluation of the peripheral smear will guide further testing, including the need for cell surface markers (flow cytometry) or bone marrow biopsy to access persistent elevations in white blood cell counts.

FURTHER READING

Guidelines and Protocols Advisory Committee, British Columbia Medical Association and British Columbia Ministry of Health Services. Iron deficiency: investigation and management. 15 June 2010. http://www.bcguidelines.ca/pdf/iron_deficiency.pdf.

Hutchison RE, McPherson RA. Hematology. In: McPherson R, Pincus M, eds. *Henry's Clinical Diagnosis and Management by Laboratory Methods.* 21st ed. Philadelphia: Saunders Elsevier; 2007;457–728.

Miller JL. Hemostasis and thrombosis. In: McPherson R, Pincus M, eds. *Henry's Clinical Diagnosis and Management by Laboratory Methods.* 21st ed. Philadelphia: Saunders Elsevier; 2007;729–788.

Nguyen A, Wahed A. Sources of errors in hematology and coagulation testing. In: Dasgupta A, Sepulveda J, eds. *Accurate Results in the Clinical Laboratory: A Guide to Error Detection and Correction.* Amsterdam, Neth.: Elsevier; 2013:305–314. http://dx.doi.org/10.1016/B978-0-12-415783-5.00019-0

Ontario Association of Medical Laboratories. Guidelines for the use of serum tests for iron deficiency. Revised February 2012. http://www.oaml.com/documents/IronDeficiencyFinalMarch2012_000.pdf.

Figure 6. Diagnostic algorithm for anemia with low MCV

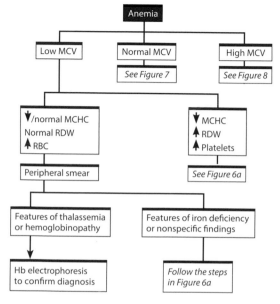

Figure 6a

(Figure 6 continued)

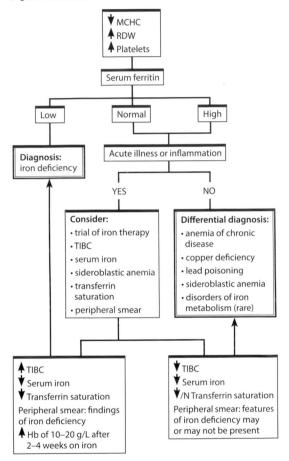

Figure 7. Diagnostic algorithm for anemia with normal MCV

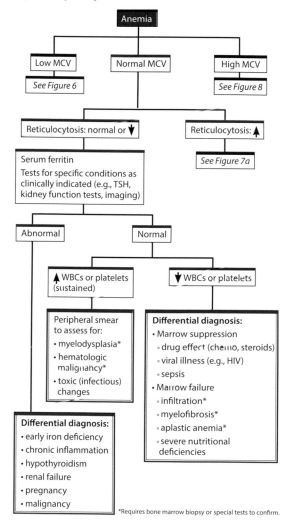

*Requires bone marrow biopsy or special tests to confirm.

Figure 7a
(Figure 7 continued)

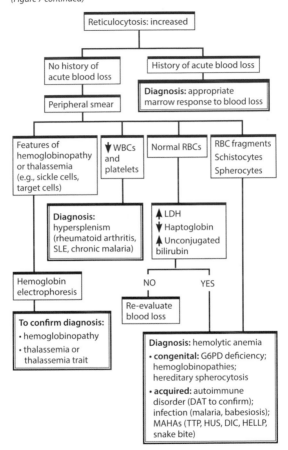

Figure 8. Diagnostic algorithm for anemia with high MCV

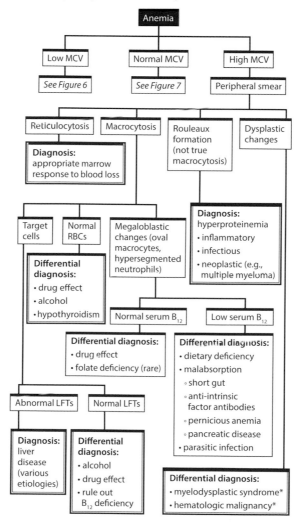

*Requires bone marrow biopsy or special tests to confirm.

Figure 9. Diagnostic algorithm for defects in primary hemostasis (mucosal bleeding)

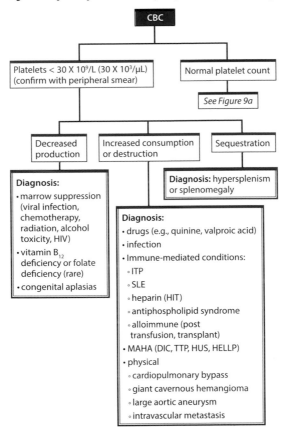

Figure 9a

(Figure 9 continued)

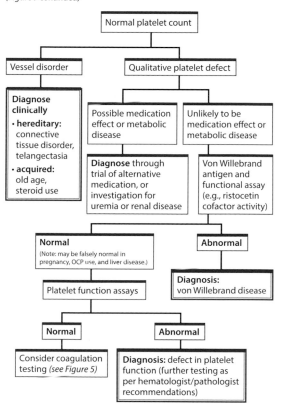

Figure 10. Diagnostic algorithm for defects in secondary hemostasis (delayed or deep tissue bleeding)

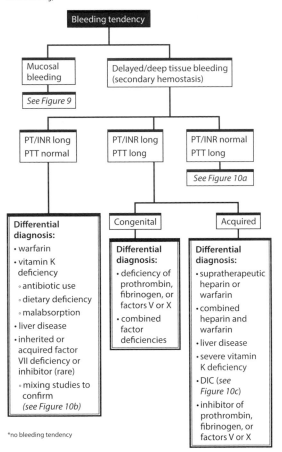

Figure 10a
(Figure 10 continued)

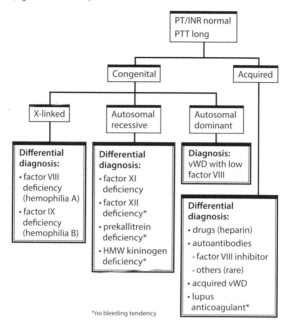

Figure 10b. Diagnostic algorithm for suspected factor deficiency or inhibitor
(Figure 10a continued)

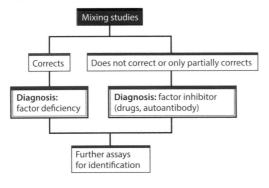

Figure 10c. Diagnostic algorithm for suspected DIC

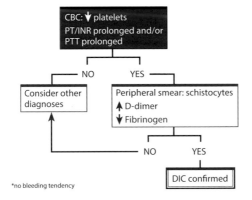

*no bleeding tendency

Figure 11. Diagnostic algorithm for unexplained thrombosis or thrombophilia

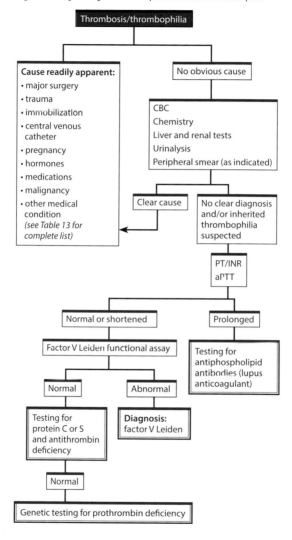

Figure 12. Diagnostic algorithm for lymphadenopathy of unclear cause

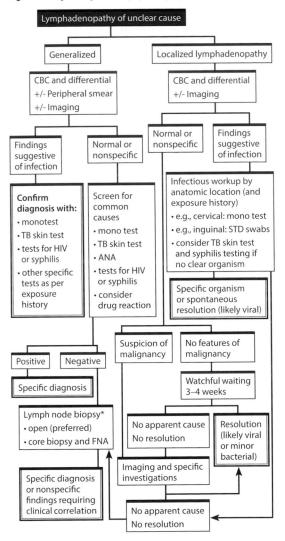

*Inform pathologist and send tissue in fresh state for culture and ancillary testing.

Figure 13. Diagnostic algorithm for splenomegaly

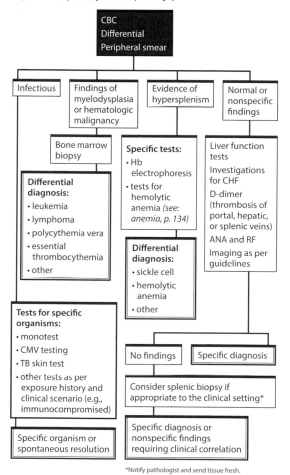

*Notify pathologist and send tissue fresh.

Intoxication and toxidromes

Dr. Leland B. Baskin

ABBREVIATIONS

6-AM	6-monoacetylmorphine	GGT	γ-glutamyltransferase
ABG	arterial blood gas	IgA	immunoglobulin A
ACh	acetylcholine	IgG	immunoglobulin G
AChE	acetylcholinesterase	LSD	lysergic acid diethylamide
AG	anion gap	MDA	3,4-methylenedioxyamphetamine
ALP	alkaline phosphatase	MDMA	3,4-methylenedioxy-*N*-methylamphetamine
ALT	alanine aminotransferase		
ASA	acetylsalicylic acid	MMDA	3-methoxy-4,5-methylenedioxyamphetamine
AST	aspartate aminotransferase		
ATP	adenosine triphosphate	NAPQI	N-acetylbenzoquinoneimine
BP	blood pressure	OG	osmolality gap
RR	respiration rate	PCP	phencyclidine
BUN	blood urea nitrogen (serum urea nitrogen)	PT	prothrombin time
		PT/INR	prothrombin time or international normalized ratio
CBC	complete blood count		
ChE	cholinesterase	RBC	red blood cell
CYP2E1	cytochrome P450 2E1	THC	tetrahydrocannabinol
eGFR	estimated glomerular filtration rate		

OVERALL APPROACH

Steps in diagnosing poisoned patients

TAKE A HISTORY, DO A PHYSICAL EXAM

Poisoning presents in a variety of fashions and can mimic numerous conditions. For this reason, as in other areas of clinical medicine, history and physical examination are initial steps that take precedence over laboratory analyses.

IDENTIFY TOXIDROMES

Toxic syndromes or "toxidromes" group clinical presentations of intoxicants by signs and symptoms.

If clinical signs and symptoms point to a toxidrome, treat the toxidrome. Laboratory analyses can help exclude or confirm the diagnosis.

For poisoned patients in general, the most effective use of laboratory analyses involves specific analyses with specific results in mind. In many cases, however, laboratory analyses do not add information useful for treatment, although they can help clarify exposure sources and prospects for recovery.

See: toxidromes, p. 178

IF NO TOXIDROME IS IDENTIFIABLE, ESTABLISH A DIFFERENTIAL DIAGNOSIS

When clinical signs and symptoms are nonspecific, a thorough history will aid in compiling a differential diagnosis.

The following initial lab assays may be useful in developing a differential diagnosis and assessing the acuity of a patient's condition[1]:

- arterial blood gas (ABG)
- cardiac and hepatic markers

- CBC
- serum electrolytes, glucose, lactate, urea
- serum osmolality

Note that:

- Assays of specific commonly used drugs for which signs and symptoms of intoxication may be nonspecific or delayed are also indicated, including assays for acetaminophen and salicylate (*see: acetaminophen, p. 192, and salicylate, p. 195*).
- For an individual with a history of taking a specific drug, either a quantitative serum or qualitative urine assay may be useful.

Emergencies

KEY PRINCIPLES

In emergency situations, history may be sparse, unobtainable, or unreliable due to coma, unexplained cardiac toxicity or acidosis, symptomatic head trauma, unexpected seizures, or multiple drug ingestion.[2]

Keep the limits of laboratory testing,[3] and the following principles, in mind:

- Therapy may need to begin before laboratory testing can identify intoxicants. Due to time constraints in emergency situations, laboratory tests do not generally help in acute diagnosis and treatment but may be useful in establishing the final diagnosis and prognosis.
- Often, you only need to identify the drug class, not the specific drug, to provide life-saving treatment.
- The cornerstones of care for overdose patients—aggressive support of ventilatory,

cardiovascular, metabolic, and neurologic functions—are mostly independent of the drugs involved.[4(p47)]

- Serum concentration provides the best quantitative assessment of a drug in the body.
- If you know the drugs involved, quantitative assessment of serial blood specimens collected over several hours is more useful than a drug screen.
- Broad toxicology screens may be useful in emergencies where obtaining a reliable history is a challenge.[4(p50)]

EMERGENCY TOXICOLOGY

Emergency toxicology (quantitative tests with turn-around times of minutes to hours) allows the timely identification or exclusion of acute intoxication by compounds that may have specific antidotes or therapies such as dialysis.

Note that:

- Quantitative blood analyses are preferred when blood concentrations of drugs drive the use of specific therapies (i.e., when they correlate with pharmacological effect).
- Serial analyses may aid in determining pharmacokinetic properties and evaluating response to therapy.

Among the most useful specific toxicologic assays are rapid quantitative analyses for[3,4(pp48,50)]:

- acetaminophen
- alcohols (ethanol, methanol, ethylene glycol)
- carbamazepine
- carbon monoxide
- digoxin
- iron

- lithium
- phenobarbital
- salicylate
- theophylline
- valproic acid

QUALITATIVE SUBSTANCE-ABUSE SCREENING

A positive qualitative substance-abuse screen means that a compound in a specified drug class is present above a specific threshold concentration, which is not necessarily toxic. Depending on the class, a positive result means that at least a typical dose was consumed within the previous 3 to 5 days. A negative result means that no compound within the specified drug class is present above the threshold for positivity. It does not imply that the drug is absent or has not been consumed.

Qualitative substance-abuse screening is usually best assessed using urine and is limited to drugs that:

- are fairly rapidly metabolized
- have a large apparent volume of distribution

The results of urine drug screens almost never change acute patient management, because urine drug concentration is not necessarily related to a drug's pharmacologic effect or the current status of the patient. Laboratories do not process these screens as a priority, which means turnaround times are longer than for quantitative analyses (hours or days).

CLINICAL PRESENTATIONS

Toxidromes

If you suspect a toxic syndrome or "toxidrome," always begin by identifying it clinically (see Table 19) and treating it.[4,5]

Table 19. Clinical features of toxic syndromes*

Syndrome	Pulse	BP	RR	Pupils	Signs and symptoms
Anticholinergic	↑	↑	N	Dil	Confusion
					Constipation without bowel sounds
					Dry skin and mucous membranes
					Fever
					Flushing
					Urinary retention
					Visual blurring
Cholinergic	↑	↑/↓	↑/N	Con	*See: cholinergic toxidrome, p. 180*
Hallucinogenic	↑/N	↑/N	N	Dil/N	Depersonalization
					Hallucinations
					Visual illusions
					Hypertension
					Psychosis
					Sensory distortion
					Tachycardia
Narcotic	N/↓	N/↓	↓	Con	Decreased consciousness
					Coma
Sedative/ hypnotic	N/↓	N/↓	N	N/Con	Confusion
					Stupor
					Coma
					Gait disturbance
					Hypothermia
					Nystagmus

Continued on p. 179

Continued from p. 178

Syndrome	Pulse	BP	RR	Pupils	Signs and symptoms
Sympathetic	↑	↑	N/↓	Dil	Diaphoresis
					Hallucinations
					Headache
					Hyperthermia
					Increased motor activity
					Psychosis
					Seizures
					Tremor
Withdrawal	↑	↑	N/↓	Dil	Abdominal cramping
					Diarrhea
					Hallucinations
					Increased motor activity
					Lacrimation
					Piloerection
					Psychosis
					Seizures
					Tremor
					Yawning

*Abbreviations in this table:
Con   constricted (miosis)
Dil   dilated (mydriasis)
N normal

Use laboratory analyses to exclude or confirm the diagnosis established clinically (see the information on specific toxidromes that follows).

ANTICHOLINERGIC TOXIDROME

KEYS TO WORKUP

Identify the toxidrome clinically (see Table 19) and treat it.

Note that the classic clinical features of the anticholinergic toxidrome are "red as a beet, dry as a bone, mad as a hatter, blind as a bat, and hot as a hare."

Common causative agents include:

- antihistamines
- antiparkinsonian agents
- phenothiazines
- tricyclic antidepressants
- *Atropa belladonna* (deadly nightshade)
- belladonna alkaloids such as atropine and scopolamine
- *Datura stramonium* (jimsonweed)

Immunoassays for specific drugs or classes of drugs of interest are not generally available. If identification is indicated (e.g., to prevent further exposure or for forensics), chromatographic analyses are usually necessary.

LAB INVESTIGATIONS

Order urine analysis for specific drugs, as indicated.

Note that the lab will determine the method to use, depending on the drug specified.

PEARLS

Sympathetic and anticholinergic toxidromes overlap. Key distinguishing features are[2]:

- anticholinergic agents cause dry skin and absent bowel sounds
- sympathomimetic agents cause diaphoresis without affecting bowel sounds

CHOLINERGIC TOXIDROME[4,6,7]

KEYS TO WORKUP

Identify the toxidrome clinically (see Table 19) and treat it.

Cholinergic toxidromes often have rapid onset of signs and symptoms, so early life-saving treatment nearly always depends on recognizing the signs and symptoms in the proper clinical setting.

Laboratory tests have little use in the acute diagnosis and treatment of cholinergic toxidromes. However, measurement of acetylcholinesterase (AChE) or butyryl ChE activity might be indicated to assess degree of intoxication and to determine prognosis, which can involve chronic neuropathic syndromes lasting days to years. Laboratory documentation of exposure to a specific intoxicant can also be useful for public health and forensic purposes (but note that intoxicants are rapidly metabolized and excreted).

The cholinergic toxidrome is caused by inhibition of AChE degradation of acetylcholine (ACh) in neural junctions, which in turn causes overstimulation of cholinergic receptors. Cholinergic receptors are either muscarinic or nicotinic; these have different functions, structures, and mechanisms of action, and are found in different locations. This means 2 types of cholinergic toxidromes can occur:

- muscarinic toxidrome (more common)
- nicotinic toxidrome

The signs and symptoms vary according to:

- the balance of the nicotinic and muscarinic effects
- the type of chemical involved
- the route of exposure

Nicotinic receptors respond more quickly than muscarinic receptors, so the nicotinic toxidrome has a faster onset.

Pupillary diameter also distinguishes these toxidromes:

- muscarinic: constricted (miosis)
- nicotinic: dilated (mydriasis)

MUSCARINIC TOXIDROME

The muscarinic toxidrome is characterized by parasympathetic postganglionic "hollow organ" hyperactivity. The breakdown that follows shows 2 mnemonics for its clinical features.

Mnemonic **dumbbels**:	Mnemonic **sludge**:
diarrhea (less frequent), diaphoresis	**s**alivation
urination (less frequent)	**l**acrimation (less frequent)
miosis (constricted or "pinpoint" pupils)	**u**rination (less frequent)
bradycardia with hypotension	**d**iarrhea (less frequent), diaphoresis
bronchoconstriction with bronchorrhea	**G**I pain
emesis	**e**mesis
lacrimation (less frequent)	
salivation	

Causative agents include:

- AChE inhibitors, such as organophosphate insecticides, and nerve agents and carbamates (most common)
- ACh
- areca (betel) nut
- carbachol
- pilocarpine
- poisonous mushrooms (*Clitocybe dealbata* and *Inocybe* spp.)

NICOTINIC TOXIDROME

The nicotinic toxidrome is characterized by sympathetic, parasympathetic, and somatic cholinergic hyperactivity. Its clinical features are (days-of-the-week mnemonic: **MTWHF**):

> **m**ydriasis
>
> **t**achycardia, tightness, tremors
>
> **w**eakness
>
> **h**ypertension, hyperglycemia
>
> **f**asciculation (most reliable sign)

Cyanosis and pallor may also be seen.

Agents known to cause this include:

- black widow spider (*Latrodectus mactans*) venom
- AChE inhibitors

- nicotine in the form of insecticides and tobacco

LAB INVESTIGATIONS

AMYLASE AND LIPASE

Order these tests to assess for pancreatitis if it is suspected clinically following organophosphate poisoning.

SERUM BUTYRYL ChE OR RBC AChE

These tests are used to approximate nerve junction concentrations and estimate degree of intoxication. These results, however, may not be valid unless pre-exposure levels are available for comparison, since normal concentrations vary widely.

Serum butyryl ChE is depressed more rapidly than RBC AChE and may remain depressed longer; however, RBC activity is thought to be a better marker for intoxication.

The following breakdown applies to both serum butyryl ChE and RBC AChE.

Cholinesterase activity (% baseline)	Degree of intoxication
> 60	none
20–60	mild
10–20	moderate
< 10	severe

ABOUT PREANALYTIC EFFECTS ON CHOLINESTERASE ACTIVITY

Numerous conditions and a few drugs can confound ChE results. Antimalarial drugs have been reported to depress RBC activity; acute infections, genetic deficiencies, liver disease, some chronic debilitating diseases, malnutrition, pregnancies, opiates, and a few other compounds depress serum activity. Some anemias and oral contraceptives depress both forms. Nephrotic syndrome has been reported to elevate serum activity.

PEARLS

AChE inhibitors may cause both muscarinic and nicotinic toxidromes: because nicotinic receptors respond faster, the nicotinic has earlier onset, but the muscarinic usually predominates (except in pediatric exposures, which more often show nicotinic signs).

The presence of both miosis and fasciculations is essentially pathognomonic for organophosphate intoxication.

Although few lab tests are useful in diagnosing the cause of cholinergic toxidromes, AChE inhibitors can affect several assays. These nonspecific findings include hyperglycemia, glycosuria, hypo- or hyperkalemia, leukocytosis, elevated creatine kinase, and decreased lipids.

HALLUCINOGENIC TOXIDROME

KEYS TO WORKUP

Identify the toxidrome clinically (see Table 19) and treat it.

Common causative agents include:

- "designer" amphetamines (MMDA, MDA and MDMA)
- cannabinoids
- lysergic acid diethylamide (LSD)
- mescaline
- phencyclidine
- psilocybin
- other, newer drugs: cathinone analogues of the amphetamines listed above (often sold as "bath salts") and synthetic cannabinoids

Lab tests can identify the particular agent involved, if identification is indicated (e.g., to prevent further exposure or for forensics).

LAB INVESTIGATIONS

URINE IMMUNOASSAYS

Use these as indicated to identify:

- phencyclidine (PCP)
- sympathomimetic amines
- tetrahydrocannabinol (THC) and other cannabinoids

SPECIFIC DRUG ANALYSES

Order these tests if clinical evidence points to other causative agents and identification is indicated.

Note that the lab will determine which test to use, depending on the drugs you specify.

PEARLS

False-positive results are possible, but very rare, for THC.

False-positive results for urine THC immunoassays are possible, depending on the assay cut-off, but highly unlikely following passive exposure to cannabis.

As a fat-soluble drug, THC is found in urine much longer than other drugs (up to 30 days or more following exposure). Serial sampling may distinguish between continuous use and abstinence.

NARCOTIC TOXIDROME

KEYS TO WORKUP

Identify the toxidrome clinically (see Table 19) and treat it.

Causative agents include:

- dextromethorphan
- diphenoxylate
- fentanyl

- opiates (codeine, morphine, oxycodone, hydrocodone, heroin)
- pentazocine
- propoxyphene

Blood assays for specific drugs or classes of drugs of interest are not generally available, but urine immunoassays for some classes are. If identification is indicated (e.g., to prevent further exposure or for forensics), order confirmatory assays. The lab will determine the best technique. Knowledge of metabolic pathways is critical to interpretation of the findings.

Note that use of the competitive opiate antagonist naloxone (Narcan) helps make the diagnosis of opiate intoxication and treats the patient as well. Naloxone rapidly (< 1 minute) blocks the μ-opioid receptors to such an extent that it may elicit a withdrawal toxidrome (*see: withdrawal toxidrome, p. 191*).

LAB INVESTIGATIONS

URINE IMMUNOASSAYS
Order these tests if you suspect opiates or opioids.

SPECIFIC DRUG ANALYSES
Order these tests if clinical evidence points to other causative agents and identification is indicated.

Note that the lab will determine which test to use, depending on the drugs you specify.

PEARLS
Urine immunoassays detect opiates up to 3 days following ingestion.

The presence of 6-monoacetylmorphine (6-AM) is conclusive evidence of heroin use: it is found in biological specimens solely due to in vivo deacetylation of heroin (3,6 diacetylmorphine).

About 10% of a codeine dose is demethylated to morphine, so ingestion of codeine and morphine result in similar metabolites in urine; however, norcodeine is specific to codeine exposure.

Poppy seeds contain both morphine and codeine.

Hydromorphone and hydrocodone are minor metabolites of morphine and codeine, respectively.

The presence of morphine does not distinguish among the ingestion of codeine, morphine, heroin, or poppy seeds. A ratio of morphine to codeine of less than 2 is consistent with codeine use.[8]

SEDATIVE/HYPNOTIC TOXIDROME

KEYS TO WORKUP
Identify the toxidrome clinically (see Table 19) and treat it.

Common causative agents include:

- barbiturates
- benzodiazepines
- opioids
- ethanol
- ethylene glycol
- isopropanol
- methanol

With the exception of alcohols, blood assays for specific drugs or classes of drugs of interest are not generally available. Available lab investigations include urine immunoassays for barbiturates and benzodiazepines, and anion gap (AG) and osmolality gap (OG). If ethanol is negative on blood assay, AG and OG are useful in pointing toward other alcohols. In that case, a screen for the common toxic alcohols is indicated. If identification is indicated (e.g., to distinguish toxic alcohols in acute cases), order gas chromatography.

LAB INVESTIGATIONS

INITIAL TESTS

Order the following as an initial panel:

- blood ethanol
- sodium (for serum AG and serum OG)
- chloride, bicarbonate (for serum AG)
- glucose, urea, and serum osmolality (for serum OG)

AG and OG can help identify causative agents (see Table 20) and concentrations (see Table 21), and obviate the need for further testing.

Note that alcoholics:

- can be asymptomatic at blood levels much higher than the stated "toxic" level
- often suffer from hypoglycemia and appear intoxicated: check glucose levels if blood ethanol is negative, and AG and OG results are unclear

Table 20. Alcohol metabolites and lab results

Alcohol	Metabolites	Lab results
Ethanol	Acetaldehyde	OG++
	Acetic acid	AG++
Ethylene glycol	Oxalic acid	AG++
		OG++
		Urine Ca oxalate crystals
		↓ Serum Ca
Isopropanol	Acetone	OG+
		Normal AG
		Serum ketones++
Methanol	Formaldehyde	AG++
	Formic acid	OG++

Table 21. Predicted osmolal gaps of toxic alcohol concentrations

Alcohol	Toxic concentration		Lethal concentration	
	mmol/L (mg/dL)	mmol/kg (= mOsm/kg)	mmol/L (mg/dL)	mmol/kg (= mOsm/kg)
Acetone	8.6 (50)	8.6	43.1 (250)	43.1
Ethanol	17.4 (80)	17.4	65.2 (300)	65.2
Ethylene glycol	4 (25)	4	8.1 (50)	8.1
Isopropanol	8.3 (50)	8.3	16.7 (100)	16.7
Methanol	7.8 (25)	7.8	25 (80)	25

For information on calculating AG and OG, see p. 292 and p. 294.

BLOOD ALCOHOLS

Order follow-up tests for blood alcohols as indicated, if the results of the initial panel are unclear and you suspect toxic alcohol intoxication (i.e., methanol, isopropanol, or ethylene glycol).

URINE IMMUNOASSAYS

Order these as follow-up tests if the results of the initial panel are unclear and you suspect poisoning from barbiturates, benzodiazepines, or opiates.

PEARLS

Most hospital laboratories use an ethanol assay that employs alcohol dehydrogenase, an enzyme specific for ethanol. This assay does not detect toxic alcohols. If blood ethanol is negative or does not account for an elevated OG, toxic alcohols are a possibility.

Alcoholics are prone to drug-induced hypoglycemia, which may present as acute intoxication although the blood ethanol is below the lethal concentration.

Hypoglycemia is seen in young children with ethanol intoxication.

SYMPATHETIC TOXIDROME

KEYS TO WORKUP
Identify the toxidrome clinically (see Table 19) and treat it.

Common causative agents include:

- caffeine
- cocaine
- PCP
- sympathomimetic amines (amphetamines, ephedrine, pseudoephedrine, phenylpropanolamine)
- theophylline

Follow up with laboratory analysis of urine, specifying immunoassays for specific drugs or classes of drugs of interest.

LAB INVESTIGATIONS

URINE IMMUNOASSAYS
Order these as clinically indicated.

RARELY INDICATED
Identification of a specific sympathomimetic amine causing a positive amphetamine screen is usually not indicated. If identification is indicated, use specific drug analyses.

PEARLS
Immunoassays for the cocaine metabolite benzoylecgonine are highly specific, so a positive result is almost always true. Immunoassays for amphetamines detect numerous drugs in the sympathomimetic amine class, including commonly used cold medications. For forensic purposes, confirmation by

another method is required; for clinical purposes, correlation with history and physical examination is most important.

A positive urine immunoassay drug screen does not necessarily mean that a toxic level of a drug is present, and should be considered presumptive unless confirmed by an appropriate alternate method. Similarly, a negative screen does not necessarily mean that a drug is absent or has not been taken by a patient, but rather that the drugs sought either are not detectable or are not present in specified concentrations.

WITHDRAWAL TOXIDROME

KEYS TO WORKUP
Identify the toxidrome clinically (see Table 19) and treat it.

This toxidrome comes from the complete cessation, after heavy use, of entities such as:

- barbiturates
- benzodiazepines
- chloral hydrate
- ethanol
- opioids
- other sedatives or hypnotics

Laboratory tests can identify the entities involved (analysis of urine with immunoassays for specific drugs or classes of drugs of interest, or blood ethanol) if exposure has occurred within the window of detection (usually 3 to 5 days).

LAB INVESTIGATIONS

BLOOD GLUCOSE
Consider ordering this test for patients who are alcoholics: alcoholics are prone to drug-induced

hypoglycemia as well as alcoholic ketoacidosis when they are starved and dehydrated.

URINE IMMUNOASSAYS AND CHROMATOGRAPHIC ANALYSIS

These will be useful in documenting prior exposure and confirming possible withdrawal when history is not available. Otherwise, they are probably not useful.

PEARLS

Diagnosis of withdrawal toxidromes requires evidence of drug use. Otherwise, they may be indistinguishable from sympathetic toxidromes.

Note that:

- Both withdrawal and sympathetic toxidromes may have hallucinations, mydriasis, seizures, and tachycardia.
- Withdrawal toxidromes usually have abdominal and gastrointestinal symptoms, but sympathetic toxidromes do not.

Specific intoxicants for which assays are available

ACETAMINOPHEN

KEYS TO WORKUP

Acetaminophen is metabolized by 3 primary pathways:

- glucuronidation
- oxidation by CYP2E1 to the hepatotoxic metabolite N-acetyl-p- benzoquinone imine (NAPQI) which is then cleared by conjugation with glutathione
- sulfation

Overdoses of acetaminophen:

- saturate the sulfation pathway and, in severe intoxication, the glucuronidation pathway[9]
- deplete the body of glutathione, allowing for accumulation of NAPQI, which binds to hepatic molecules and causes hepatocellular necrosis

Signs and symptoms of hepatotoxicity[9,10]:

- usually require at least 24 to 72 hours to manifest
- may initially present as nausea and vomiting, lethargy, and pallor, with evolving liver enlargement and tenderness, and elevated PT and AST
- progress to hepatic encephalopathy, lactic acidosis, renal failure, and death

The normal plasma half-life of acetaminophen is 1 to 3 hours, but is elevated in overdose. A therapeutic dose of acetaminophen is 10 to 15 mg/kg; acute toxicity occurs at doses > 150 mg/kg.

Delayed clearance of acetaminophen is considered the most accurate method for predicting hepatotoxicity. The Rumack-Matthew nomogram[11] is used to assess the risk of hepatotoxicity. It assumes a maximum concentration of 1324 μmol/L (200 μg/mL) at 4 hours post consumption with first order decay and a plasma half-life ($t_{1/2}$) of 4 hours.

This is represented mathematically as:

$$C\,(\mu mol/L) = e^{(-0.17329\,\times\,t\,+\,7.8816)} \quad \text{SI units}$$

$$C\,(\mu g/mL) = e^{(-0.17329\,\times\,t\,+\,5.9915)} \quad \text{conventional units}$$

where t is in hours

Since the exact time of consumption is generally not known, a better method for estimating hepatotoxicity is to estimate $t_{1/2}$ based on

2 measurements at least 2 hours apart using the following equation:

$$\text{Plasma half-life } (t_{1/2}, \text{hrs}) = 0.693 \times \frac{\ln(C2/C1)}{(t2 - t1)}$$

where *C1* and *C2* are concentrations measured at times *t1* and *t2* (hrs), respectively

Hepatotoxicity is assumed at $t_{1/2}$ greater than 4 hours.

LAB INVESTIGATIONS

SERUM ACETAMINOPHEN

Order this as an initial test if you suspect acetaminophen poisoning, but note that the results can only be interpreted if the specimen was collected more than 4 hours after consumption.

If concentration is in the toxic range, repeat this test every 12 hours until a subtoxic concentration is reached.

Note that serum acetaminophen may be measured by colour test, chromatography, or immunoassay.

FOLLOW-UP TESTS

If the serum acetaminophen results are high, assess for liver and renal injury with:

- ALP, ALT, AST, indirect and direct bilirubin, GGT, PT/INR
- creatinine/eGFR

If AST is elevated, repeat ALT, PT/INR, and creatinine every 12 hours until results stabilize and the serum acetaminophen concentration is subtoxic.

Note that the following may also help assess liver and renal damage and determine prognosis:

- glucose
- electrolytes

- lactate
- phosphate
- pH

PEARLS

Susceptibility to hepatic intoxication varies widely across populations. Conditions that increase the risk of toxicity include[4(p181)]:

- alcoholism
- chronic ingestion of drugs that induce hepatic microsomal enzymes such as isoniazid and anticonvulsants
- conditions with depleted glutathione such as starvation

Acute intoxication has been reported after normal doses of acetaminophen in individuals with sub-clinical liver disease.

Careful history taking is crucial: patients who present early exhibit no specific signs or symptoms.

Serum acetaminophen analysis is recommended as cost effective in all cases of suspected poisoning, since acetaminophen is widely available and poisoning is initially asymptomatic, has significant morbidity, and is effectively treatable.

SALICYLATE[4,10,12]

KEYS TO WORKUP

Salicylate is found in a number of products but acute intoxication is mainly due to:

- aspirin (acetylsalicylic acid, ASA)
- skin care products

Salicylate has numerous pharmacologic effects, but acute toxicity results from uncoupling of oxidative phosphorylation leading to decreased adenosine triphosphate (ATP) production.

Acute signs and symptoms may be related to stimulation of the respiratory centre of the brain leading to hyperpnea and respiratory alkalosis, which is accompanied or followed by metabolic acidosis.

Presenting signs and symptoms may include:

- abdominal pain
- nausea, vomiting, and hematemesis
- hyperthermia, possibly accompanied by rhabdomyolysis and seizures
- hypokalemia
- mental status changes, ranging from agitation and seizures to lethargy, central nervous system depression, and coma
- tinnitus

Acute intoxication occurs with doses greater than 150 mg/kg. To estimate a patient's total dose, find out the approximate number and content of the tablets ingested, and the patient's weight. For example:

- ingested tablets: 40 tablets containing 325 mg each
- patient weight: 70 kg (154 lb)
- total dose: about 185 mg/kg

Toxicity occurs at serum salicylate concentration > 2.18 mmol/L (300 µg/L) with increased risk of death at concentration > 4.36 mmol/L (600 µg/L).

Peak ASA levels usually occur about 2 hours after ingestion, but may be delayed with enteric-coated tablets or massive doses. The plasma half-life of salicylic acid is dose dependent, varying from 2 to 19 hours.

Salicylate intoxication classically results in respiratory alkalosis with metabolic acidosis with an elevated AG. High doses may cause hemorrhage, nausea and vomiting, and seizures. Chronic use may lead to salicylism, which is usually associated with dizziness, dimmed vision, confusion, headache, and tinnitus.

LAB INVESTIGATIONS

SERUM SALICYLATE

Serum salicylate should be measured as soon as a clinical suspicion arises. If the concentration is elevated:

- measure it every 2 hours until it peaks
- then, every 4 to 6 hours until it reaches a subtoxic concentration[10]

It may be measured by a colour test, chromatography, or immunoassays.

OTHER TESTS

The following tests help determine the degree of toxicity, once salicylate intoxication is confirmed:

- electrolytes
- ABG
- glucose
- urea/BUN and creatinine/eGFR
- AST, ALT, and PT/INR

Consider measuring ethanol and acetaminophen if a patient's history is unclear.

INTERPRETATION: ABG

Evaluation of ABG with pH and Pco_2 allows the classification of patient status for acidosis versus alkalosis, and metabolic versus respiratory etiologies (see Table 22).

This is important since:

- CNS depressants and narcotics are associated with respiratory acidosis.

- Toxic alcohols are associated with metabolic acidosis.
- Salicylate intoxication causes respiratory alkalosis initially and is followed by compensatory metabolic acidosis.

Table 22. Interpretation of arterial blood gas results

Condition	Metabolic	Respiratory
Acidosis pH < 7.4	$[HCO_3^-] < 24$ mmol/L* ($Pco_2 < 40$ mm Hg) Ethylene glycol Methanolali Salicylate (late)	$[HCO_3^-] > 24$ mmol/L* ($Pco_2 > 40$ mm Hg) CNS depressants Opioids
Alkalosis pH ≈ 7.4	$Pco_2 > 40$ mm Hg ($[HCO_3^-] > 24$ mmol/L*)	$Pco_2 < 40$ mm Hg ($[HCO_3^-] < 24$ mmol/L*) Salicylate (early)

*24 mEq/L

PEARLS

Since signs and symptoms appear early, an alert asymptomatic patient who denies salicylate ingestion is unlikely to warrant a serum salicylate measurement.

Salicylate may be measured by enzymatic and immunoassay methods. If the results of one method don't match the clinical presentation and history, use another method. This reduces the chance of false results from an interference.

REFERENCES

1 Flomenbaum NE, Goldfrank LR, Hoffman RS, Howland MA, Lewin NA, Nelson LS. Principles of managing the poisoned or overdosed patient. In: Flomenbaum NE, Howland MA, Goldfrank LR, Lewin NA, Hoffman RS, Lewis SN, eds. *Goldfrank's Toxicologic Emergencies.* 8th ed. New York, NY: McGraw-Hill; 2006:42–50.

2 Wolf LR. *Overdoses and Poisoning: Physiological Responses and Drug Testing in the Emergency Department Patient.* Washington, DC: Therapeutic Drug Monitoring and Toxicology, American Association for Clinical Chemistry; 1997:231–247.

3   Wu AHB, McKay C, Broussard LA, et al. National Academy of Clinical Biochemistry Laboratory Medicine practice guidelines: recommendations for the use of laboratory tests to support poisoned patients who present to the emergency department. *Clin Chem.* 2003;49(3):357–379. http://dx.doi.org/10.1373/49.3.357. Medline:12600948

4   Ellenhorn MJ. *Ellenhorn's Medical Toxicology: Diagnosis and Treatment of Human Poisoning.* 2nd ed. Baltimore, MD: Williams and Wilkins; 1997.

5   Flomenbaum NE, Goldfrank LR, Hoffman RS, Howland MA, Lewin NA, Nelson LS. Initial evaluation of the patient: vital signs and toxic syndromes. In: Flomenbaum NE, Howland MA, Goldfrank LR, Lewin NA, Hoffman RS, Lewis SN, eds. *Goldfrank's Toxicologic Emergencies.* 8th ed. New York, NY: McGraw-Hill; 2006:37–41.

6   Auf der Heide E. Cholinesterase inhibitors: including pesticides and chemical warfare nerve agents. In: *Case Studies in Environmental Medicine.* Atlanta, GA: Agency for Toxic Substances and Disease Registry; 2007:1–153. http://www.atsdr.cdc.gov/csem/cholinesterase/docs/cholinesterase.pdf

7   Clark, RF. Insecticides: organic phosphorus compounds and carbamates. In: Flomenbaum NE, Howland MA, Goldfrank LR, Lewin NA, Hoffman RS, Lewis SN, eds. *Goldfrank's Toxicologic Emergencies.* 8th ed. New York, NY: McGraw-Hill; 2006:1497–1512.

8   Shults TF. *The Medical Review Officer Handbook.* 9th ed. Research Triangle Park, NC: Quadrangle Research LLC; 2009:267.

9   Hendrickson RG, Bizovi KE. Acetaminophen. In: Flomenbaum NE, Howland MA, Goldfrank LR, Lewin NA, Hoffman RS, Lewis SN, eds. *Goldfrank's Toxicologic Emergencies.* 8th ed. New York, NY: McGraw-Hill; 2006:523–543.

10 Yu H-Y E, Magnani B. Over-the-counter analgesics. In: Magnani B, Bissell MG, Kwong TC, Wu AHB, eds. *Clinical Toxicology Testing: A Guide for Laboratory Professionals.* Northfield, IL: CAP Press; 2012:179–187.

11 Rumack BH, Matthew H. Acetaminophen poisoning and toxicity. *Pediatrics.* 1975;55:871–876. Medline:1134886

12 Flomenbaum NE. Salicylates. In: Flomenbaum NE, Howland MA, Goldfrank LR, Lewin NA, Hoffman RS, Lewis SN, eds. *Goldfrank's Toxicologic Emergencies.* 8th ed. New York, NY: McGraw-Hill; 2006:550–564.

FURTHER READING

Alter D, Dufour DR. Anion gap: a review. *ASCP Case Reports: Clinical Chemistry.* Chicago, IL: American Society for Clinical Pathology; 2013.

Baskin LB, Orsulak PJ. Toxicology and substance abuse testing. In: McKenna RW, Keffer JH. *Handbook of Clinical Pathology.* 2nd ed. Chicago, IL: American Society of Clinical Pathologists; 2000:245–254.

Levine B, ed. *Principles of Forensic Toxicology.* 3rd ed. Washington, DC: AACC Press; 2010.

Perrone J. Iron. In: Flomenbaum NE, Howland MA, Goldfrank LR, Lewin NA, Hoffman RS, Lewis SN, eds. *Goldfrank's Toxicologic Emergencies.* 8th ed. New York, NY: McGraw-Hill; 2006:629–640.

Porter WH. Clinical toxicology. In: Burtis CA, Ashwood ER, Bruns DE, eds. *Tietz Textbook of Clinical Chemistry and Molecular Diagnostics.* 4th ed. St. Louis, MO: Elsevier Saunders; 2006:chap 34.

Rainey PM. Laboratory principles. In: Flomenbaum NE, Howland MA, Goldfrank LR, Lewin NA, Hoffman RS, Lewis SN, eds. *Goldfrank's Toxicologic Emergencies.* 8th ed. New York, NY: McGraw-Hill; 2006:88–108.

Musculoskeletal system

Dr. Christopher Naugler

ABBREVIATIONS

AChR	acetylcholine receptor	GGT	γ-glutamyltransferase
ALP	alkaline phosphatase	HbA$_{1c}$	glycated hemoglobin
AlT	alanine aminotransferase	HIV	human immunodeficiency virus
ANA	antinuclear antibodies	HSV	herpes simplex virus
anti-CCP	cyclic citrullinated polypeptide antibody	PT/INR	prothrombin time or international normalized ratio
AST	aspartate aminotransferase	RF	rheumatoid factor
CBC	complete blood count	SLE	systemic lupus erythematosus
CK	creatine kinase	T$_3$	triiodothyronine
CRP	C-reactive protein	T$_4$	thyroxine
CSF	cerebrospinal fluid	TSH	thyroid-stimulating hormone (thyrotropin)
ENA	extractable nuclear antigen		
ESR	erythrocyte sedimentation rate	WBC	white blood cell

OVERALL APPROACH

Table 23 gives some commonly used laboratory tests in the workup of muscle and joint pain.

These tests are often better at ruling out a diagnosis than confirming a diagnosis: many of them are nonspecific and have significant positivity rates in the healthy general population.

Order them judiciously, and never as screening tests.

In addition, do not order HLA-B27 as a screening test: patients positive for HLA-B27, but without a family history of ankylosing spondylitis, have only a 2% chance of developing this disorder.

Table 23. Some commonly ordered laboratory tests in the evaluation of muscle and joint pain

Test	Purpose
Antinuclear antibodies (ANA)	Diagnosis of systemic lupus erythematosus (SLE), drug-induced lupus, Sjögren syndrome, scleroderma, polymyositis, dermatomyositis, and autoimmune hepatitis
C-reactive protein (preferred) or erythrocyte sedimentation rate (ESR)	Measure of the presence and severity of inflammation
Complete blood count (CBC)	Detection of anemia or white blood cell abnormalities Lymphopenia and thrombocytopenia may indicate the presence of SLE
Creatine kinase (CK)	Diagnosis of polymyositis or statin-induced myopathy
Rheumatoid factor (RF)	Diagnosis of rheumatoid arthritis.
Thyroid-stimulating hormone (TSH)	Diagnosis of thyroid disease
Urinalysis	Hematuria and proteinuria may indicate the presence of renal involvement, and especially of SLE

DISORDERS AND CLINICAL PRESENTATIONS

FIBROMYALGIA

KEYS TO WORKUP

The diagnosis of fibromyalgia is clinical, based on the presence of compatible signs and symptoms.

A few basic laboratory tests help rule out alternative diagnoses.

LAB INVESTIGATIONS

If you suspect fibromyalgia, order the following tests as a panel:

- C-reactive protein (CRP)
- CBC
- CK
- TSH

Note that all these tests should have normal results in fibromyalgia.

PEARLS

CRP is a more sensitive test than ESR for detecting systemic inflammation.

GUILLAIN-BARRÉ SYNDROME/ PERIPHERAL NEUROPATHY

KEYS TO WORKUP

The diagnosis of Guillain-Barré syndrome is clinical, based on the presence of compatible signs and symptoms. Note that the following workup could also apply to peripheral-neuropathy testing where the diagnosis is unclear.

A few basic laboratory tests help rule out alternative diagnoses, such as diabetes, liver dysfunction, and thyroid disorders. In rare cases, herpes simplex virus (HSV) and HIV can produce signs and symptoms similar to Guillain-Barré syndrome.

LAB INVESTIGATIONS

TESTS FOR GUILLAIN-BARRÉ SYNDROME

If you suspect Guillain-Barré syndrome, order the following tests as a panel:

- CRP
- CBC

- CK
- HbA$_{1c}$
- liver function tests: ALT, ALP, AST, indirect and direct bilirubin, GGT, PT/INR
- serum protein electrophoresis
- TSH

Note that all these tests should have normal results in Guillain-Barré syndrome and peripheral neuropathy.

TESTS FOR HSV AND HIV (RARELY INDICATED)

Consider testing for HSV and HIV in cases difficult to diagnose, if history and presentation suggest these causes as possibilities.

- HSV: viral culture or antigen detection test, if fresh sores are present
- HIV: serology

PEARLS

CRP is a more sensitive test than ESR for detecting systemic inflammation.

Further specific workup for Guillain-Barré syndrome may involve nerve conduction studies and lumbar puncture to look for an elevated CSF protein level. Nerve conduction studies are also useful in the workup of peripheral neuropathy.

MONOARTHRITIS, ACUTE

KEYS TO WORKUP

The diagnosis of acute monoarthritis is primarily clinical, based on the presence of compatible signs and symptoms.

If clinical evidence points to septic arthritis, or if the diagnosis is unclear, synovial fluid analysis is indicated.

LAB INVESTIGATIONS

STAT TESTS OF SYNOVIAL FLUID

If you suspect septic arthritis or need to clarify a diagnosis, perform arthrocentesis on the affected joint.

Order stat testing of the synovial fluid as follows:

- cell count
- crystal analysis
- culture
- Gram stain

A synovial fluid WBC count greater than $2 \times 10^9/L$ (2000 WBC/mm^3) suggests inflammation; counts greater than $50 \times 10^9/L$ (50 000 WBC/ mm^3) are usually seen with infection but the values may overlap in these entities. Cultures are positive in half of nongonococcal infections. If gonococcal infection is suspected, then pharyngeal, urethral, cervical, and rectal cultures should be performed.

STAT COLLECTION FOR BLOOD CULTURE

If you suspect septic arthritis, draw blood and order a stat collection for blood culture, in addition to the tests on synovial fluid.

OTHER TESTS

Depending on history and physical findings, test for:

- HIV antibodies
- Lyme disease antibodies

NOT RECOMMENDED

Other tests such as RF, ANA, and uric acid are not useful in the assessment of acute monoarthritis.

MUSCLE PAIN

KEYS TO WORKUP

History and physical examination should guide any laboratory investigations.

Statin-induced myopathy and thyroid disease are especially important entities to consider.

If a patient does not take statins and has no clinical signs of thyroid disorder, consider electrolyte imbalance as a cause.

LAB INVESTIGATIONS

CK

Order this test for patients receiving statin medications to rule out statin-induced myopathy.

TESTS FOR THYROID DISORDERS

Use the following tests to rule out thyroid disease (hyper- and hypothyroidism):

- TSH: start with this test, which is the single best initial test for thyroid disorders
- TSH with T_4: follow up with this test if the initial TSH is elevated, to confirm a diagnosis of hypothyroidism
- T_4: follow up with this test if the TSH is suppressed to confirm hyperthyroidism
- T_3: this is rarely indicated, and is useful only when TSH is suppressed but free T_4 is normal (a pattern known as T_3 toxicosis)

See: thyroid disorders, p. 33

ELECTROLYTES, MAGNESIUM, CALCIUM

Order these tests as a panel, as clinically indicated, to rule out electrolyte disturbances.

MYASTHENIA GRAVIS

KEYS TO WORKUP

The diagnosis of myasthenia gravis is primarily clinical, based on the presence of compatible signs and symptoms. The diagnosis is supported by the presence of acetylcholine receptor antibodies (AChR antibodies) and is generally confirmed by a drug challenge test. In all cases, it is important to rule out hyper- and hypothyroidism.

LAB INVESTIGATIONS

AChR ANTIBODY AND CLINICAL TENSILON TESTING

As clinically indicated, rule out myasthenia gravis by testing for acetylcholine receptor antibody (AChR antibody) and with Tensilon testing.

AChR antibody testing has:

- 50% sensitivity when myasthenia gravis is confined to the eyes
- 80% sensitivity when myasthenia gravis is generalized

TESTS FOR THYROID DISORDERS

Use the following tests to rule out thyroid disease (hyper- and hypothyroidism):

- TSH: start with this test, which is the single best initial test for thyroid disorders
- TSH with T_4: follow up with this test if the initial TSH is elevated, to confirm a diagnosis of hypothyroidism
- T_4: follow up with this test if the TSH is suppressed to confirm hyperthyroidism
- T_3: this is rarely indicated, and is useful only when TSH is suppressed but free T_4 is normal (a pattern known as T_3 toxicosis)

See: thyroid disorders, p. 33

POLYARTHRITIS

KEYS TO WORKUP

There are no definitive rheumatologic laboratory tests. History and physical examination should guide decisions about testing, and the clinical situation is crucial to interpreting lab results.

Note that:

- Many rheumatologic laboratory tests are positive in a significant portion of healthy individuals.
- Some basic laboratory tests such as a CBC, CRP, and urinalysis may yield very useful findings (see Table 23).

LAB INVESTIGATIONS

TESTS FOR RHEUMATOID ARTHRITIS

If you suspect rheumatoid arthritis, order the following tests as a panel:

- CRP
- RF: note that this has a poor sensitivity and specificity

If available, also consider ordering:

- cyclic citrullinated polypeptide antibody (anti-CCP): this is more specific than rheumatoid factor, but is generally less available

TESTS FOR SLE

If you suspect SLE, order the following tests as a panel:

- ANA
- urinalysis: to rule out renal involvement

ANA interpretation is complex: see Table 24 for the major patterns.

If a positive ANA pattern is detected, consider follow-up testing for extractable nuclear antigens (ENA), which may point more specifically to a clinical entity (see Table 25).

Table 24. Interpretation of ANA patterns

Pattern	Associated conditions
Centromere pattern (peripheral)	CREST syndrome (calcinosis, Raynaud syndrome, esophageal dysmotility, sclerodactyly, telangiectasia)
	Scleroderma
Homogenous (diffuse)	Mixed connective tissue disease
	SLE
Nucleolar	Polymyositis
	Scleroderma
Speckled	Mixed connective tissue disease
	Polymyositis
	Rheumatoid arthritis
	Scleroderma
	Sjögren syndrome
	SLE

Table 25. Interpretation of ENA patterns

Antigen	Conditions associated with the presence of antibodies
Jo-1	Polymyositis
	Dermatomyositis
nRNP	Mixed connective tissue disease
	SLE
Scl-70	Scleroderma
Sm	SLE
SSA-60/Ro	Sjögren syndrome
	SLE
	Note: false positives are associated with parasitic infections
SSB/La	Rheumatoid arthritis
	Scleroderma
	Sjögren syndrome
	SLE

Note: the majority of these tests have poor sensitivities for the associated conditions.

FURTHER READING

Funovits J, Aletaha D, Bykerk V, et al. The 2010 American College of Rheumatology/European League Against Rheumatism classification criteria for rheumatoid arthritis: methodological report phase I. *Ann Rheum Dis*. 2010;69(9):1589–1595. .

Phan TG, Wong RCW, Adelstein S. Autoantibodies to extractable nuclear antigens: making detection and interpretation more meaningful. *Clin Diagn Lab Immunol*. 2002;9(1):1–7. Medline:11777822

Mies Richie A, Francis ML. Diagnostic approach to polyarticular joint pain. *Am Fam Physician*. 2003;68(6):1151–1160. Medline:14524403

Siva C, Velazquez C, Mody A, Brasington R. Diagnosing acute monoarthritis in adults: a practical approach for the family physician. *Am Fam Physician*. 2003;68(1):83–90. Medline:12887114

Neuropsychiatry

Dr. Davinder Sidhu

ABBREVIATIONS

ABG	arterial blood gas	hCG	human chorionic gonadotropin
AChR	antibody acetylcholine receptor antibody	LOC	level of consciousness
		MAOI	monoamine oxidase inhibitor
ALP	alkaline phosphatase	PT/INR	prothrombin time or international normalized ratio
ALT	alanine aminotransferase		
AST	aspartate aminotransferase	RPR	rapid plasma reagin
CBC	complete blood count	SNRI	serotonin/norepinephrine reuptake inhibitor
CK	creatine kinase		
CNS	central nervous system	SSRI	selective serotonin reuptake inhibitor
CRP	C-reactive protein		
CSF	cerebrospinal fluid	T_3	triiodothyronine
DIC	disseminated intravascular coagulation	T_4	thyroxine
		TCA	tricyclic antidepressant
ECG	electrocardiogram	TIA	transient ischemic attack
ESR	erythrocyte sedimentation rate	TSH	thyroid-stimulating hormone (thyrotropin)
GABA	γ-aminobutyric acid		
GGT	γ-glutamyltransferase	TTP	thrombotic thrombocytopenic purpura
HbA_{1c}	glycated hemoglobin		

OVERALL APPROACH

Laboratory testing is useful in the workup of many neurologic and psychiatric illnesses.

In the diagnosis of any psychiatric illness, testing helps rule out underlying medical conditions, exogenous medications, substance abuse, and toxidromes, which may induce behavioural changes that mimic true psychological pathology.

In organic neurologic diseases, laboratory tests can help to distinguish several common causes, including infections, autoimmune disease, and side effects from specific medications or toxins.

If you suspect a toxidrome:

- Identify the toxidrome clinically and treat it.
- Use lab tests to rule in or out specific drugs related to the toxidrome.
- If no toxidrome can be identified clinically, establish a differential diagnosis and consider tests to identify other substances.

To rule out mood alteration from a toxidrome, consider:

- blood alcohol levels
- liver enzymes
- urine drug screen

See: intoxication and toxidromes, p. 173

DISORDERS AND CLINICAL PRESENTATIONS

Psychiatric disorders

ANXIETY

KEYS TO WORKUP
Common medical conditions associated with anxiety include:

- heart disease
- asthma
- diabetes
- thyroid disorders
- drug abuse or withdrawal (particularly withdrawal from antianxiety medications such as benzodiazepines)
- alcohol withdrawal
- certain neuroendocrine tumours

Anxiety may also develop as a side effect to certain medications, including:

- asthma medications (e.g., albuterol)
- antihypertensives (e.g., methyldopa)
- hormones (e.g., oral contraceptives)
- steroids (e.g., cortisone, dexamethasone, prednisone)
- amphetamine compounds (e.g., Benzedrine, Dexedrine, Ritalin)
- thyroid medications (e.g., Synthroid)
- other medicines (e.g., levodopa, phenytoin, quinidine)

Depending on the severity of the clinical presentation, consider tests to rule out medication side effects and thyroid disorders.

Base decisions about further investigations on clinical findings for underlying medical conditions.

LAB INVESTIGATIONS

TESTS FOR THYROID DISORDERS

As clinically indicated, use the following tests to rule out thyroid disease (hyper- and hypothyroidism):

- TSH: start with this test, which is the single best initial test for thyroid disorders

- TSH with T_4: follow up with this test if the initial TSH is elevated, to confirm a diagnosis of hypothyroidism
- T_4: follow up with this test if the initial TSH is suppressed to confirm hyperthyroidism
- T_3: this is rarely indicated, and is useful only when TSH is suppressed but free T_4 is normal (a pattern known as T_3 toxicosis)

See: thyroid disorders, p. 33

DEMENTIA AND COGNITIVE IMPAIRMENT

KEYS TO WORKUP

Most progressive dementias have organic causes that include Alzheimer disease, Lewy body dementia, vascular dementia, frontotemporal dementias, and infection. Other causes include genetic diseases such as Huntington disease, which require genetic testing to diagnose. Remember that depression is a common mimicker of cognitive impairment and must always be ruled out.

Laboratory testing can be very useful for ruling out reversible causes of dementia, such as drugs (common) and metabolic disorders.

Metabolic abnormalities contribute to cognitive dysfunction in 1% to 2% of cases. Among these, the most common are:

- diabetes
- renal failure
- hyponatremia
- folate deficiency (rare)
- vitamin B_{12} deficiency
- hyperthyroidism

Depending on patient history, other causes such as hypoxia, congestive heart failure, and neoplasms must be considered.

LAB INVESTIGATIONS

CBC

Order this test as part of your initial workup.

This test can:

- rule out vitamin B_{12} and folate deficiency (megaloblastoid changes in cells)
- suggest anemia of chronic disease (from thyroid or renal problems)
- rule out infection (white blood cell increases)

URINE DRUG SCREEN

Order this test if you suspect drugs are involved, based on clinical symptoms and patient drug history.

TESTS FOR HYPERTHYROIDISM

To rule out hyperthyroidism:

- Start with TSH, which is the single best initial test for thyroid disorders.
- Follow up with T_4 if the initial TSH is suppressed.

Note that T_3 is rarely indicated, and is useful only when TSH is suppressed but free T_4 is normal (a pattern known as T_3-toxicosis).

See: hyperthyroidism, p. 33

RENAL FUNCTION TESTS

Measure creatinine/eGFR to ensure proper excretion of toxic metabolites, which may accumulate and mimic, or contribute to, cognitive decline.

This is particularly important in the elderly, who may be on polypharmacy treatment.

ELECTROLYTES

Order this test as clinically indicated.

Electrolytic balances can critically affect osmotic gradients, neuromuscular transmission, and acid-base balances. Imbalance can signal metabolic derangements, which can affect cognitive function (hyper- or hypoglycemia showing shifts in K^+ cations). Metabolic derangements can also directly contribute to cognitive dysfunction by shifting osmotic balances in tissues and causing edema in the brain (hyper- or hyponatremia).

LIVER FUNCTION TESTS

Order liver function tests as clinically indicated. These tests may include ALP, ALT, AST, indirect and direct bilirubin, GGT, and PT/INR.

Liver function is important in detoxification and excretion of several metabolic pathways. Interruption of these detoxification pathways can result in accumulation of metabolites that affect cognitive function. Liver failure with the development of ascites can lead to abdominal fluid buildup and a nidus for chronic bacterial infection to further drive cognitive decline.

RPR (SYPHILIS)

Order a rapid plasma reagin (RPR) test as clinically indicated.

Tertiary syphilis can present as neurosyphilis in 6.5% of untreated infections within 3 to 15 years following primary infection. These patients present with neuromuscular deficits and cognitive decline, along with disinhibition, apathy, and seizure.

GLUCOSE

Order this test as clinically indicated.

Diabetic neuropathy can affect sensation and fine motor control in longstanding diabetics and mimic functional impairments of other CNS disease. Hypoglycemia can be related to seizure, mood alteration, and violence, similar to that noted in many delirious and demented patients.

NOT RECOMMENDED

Tests for vitamin B_{12} deficiency have low clinical yield. Although B_{12} deficiency is associated with dementia, no good evidence shows that B_{12} replacement reverses cognitive impairment.

Tests for folate deficiency also have low clinical yield. Folate deficiency is rare in Canada since universal flour supplementation began several decades ago. Note, however, that folate testing may still make sense for refugees and new immigrants to Canada, and for patients with chronic malabsorptive syndromes (e.g., celiac disease, Crohn disease).

DEPRESSION

KEYS TO WORKUP

Symptoms of depression have a long differential. Diagnosis of a primary psychiatric cause requires ruling out other causes: underlying medical conditions, medications, toxins, and drugs.

Common medical conditions associated with depression include:

- alcohol withdrawal
- anemia
- asthma
- diabetes
- drug abuse or drug withdrawal (particularly withdrawal from antianxiety medications such as benzodiazepines)
- heart disease
- certain neuroendocrine tumours and malignancies
- thyroid disorders

Note that some medications may be associated with depression (see the breakdown that follows). Consider patient drug history and urine drug screen for exogenous causes.

Category	Examples	Common brand names
Antidepressants	Monoamine oxidase inhibitors (MAOIs)	Nardil
		Parnate
	Selective serotonin reuptake inhibitors (SSRIs)	Paxil
		Prozac
	Serotonin/norepinephrine reuptake inhibitors (SNRIs)	Cymbalta
		Effexor
		Pristiq
	Tricyclic antidepressants (TCAs)	Elavil
		Pamelor
Antirejection medications	Cyclosporine	Neoral
Antispastic medications	Baclofen (GABA receptor agonists)	Lioresal
Corticosteroids	Hydrocortisone	Azmacort
	Prednisone	Flonase
	Triamcinolone	Flovent
		Nasacort
		Nasonex
Parkinson medications	Levodopa	Artane
	Trihexyphenidyl	Sinemet
Thyroid medications	Levothyroxine	Synthroid

LAB INVESTIGATIONS

CBC

Use this test as clinically indicated, to assess for anemia.

See: anemia, p. 134

CALCIUM

Consider this test if patients have a history of hypercalcemia or malignancy.

TESTS FOR THYROID DISORDERS

As clinically indicated, use the following tests to rule out thyroid disease (hyper- and hypothyroidism):

- TSH: start with this test, which is the single best initial test for thyroid disorders
- TSH with T_4: follow up with this test if the initial TSH is elevated, to confirm a diagnosis of hypothyroidism
- T_4: follow up with this test if the initial TSH is suppressed to confirm hyperthyroidism
- T_3: this is rarely indicated, and is useful only when TSH is suppressed but free T_4 is normal (a pattern known as T_3-toxicosis)

See: thyroid disorders, p. 33

URINE DRUG SCREEN

Order this test as clinically indicated, based on signs and symptoms, and patient drug history.

Note that urine drug screens:

- can provide comprehensive testing for many commonly abused street and prescription drugs, if you are uncertain of the drugs involved
- can test for specific drugs, if you suspect specific drugs are involved

MANIA AND HYPOMANIA

KEYS TO WORKUP

Diagnosing mania and hypomania commonly requires distinguishing elevated mood disorders from substance abuse disorders.

LAB INVESTIGATIONS

URINE DRUG SCREEN

Order this test as clinically indicated, based on signs and symptoms, and patient drug history.

Note that urine drug screens:

- can provide comprehensive testing for many commonly abused street and prescription drugs, if you are uncertain of the drugs involved
- can test for specific drugs, if you suspect specific drugs are involved

Neurological disorders

ALTERED LEVELS OF CONSCIOUSNESS

KEYS TO WORKUP

To diagnose fluctuating level of consciousness (LOC), first rule out traumatic, vascular, and structural causes by clinical examination and imaging. Laboratory testing can then help to distinguish metabolic, drug, and infectious causes (meningitis or encephalitis).

Common metabolic changes that can cause cognitive impairment include:

- hypoxia
- hypercapnia
- hyper- or hypokalemia
- hyper- or hyponatremia
- hyper- or hypocalcemia

Other medical conditions can include sepsis, disseminated intravascular coagulation (DIC), thrombotic thrombocytopenic purpura (TTP), and secondary hypertension.

Drugs that affect cognitive function include:

- opiates
- alcohol
- barbiturates
- polypharmacy reactions

Use laboratory investigations to rule out:

- first, drug-induced causes
- next, metabolic causes
- then, infectious causes

LAB INVESTIGATIONS

INITIAL PANEL

Begin with these tests:

- blood alcohol
- glucose
- urine drug screen (sedatives, barbiturates)

ABG AND ELECTROLYTES

Order tests for arterial blood gas (ABG) and electrolytes if the initial panel is inconclusive.

These test for metabolic abnormalities (Na, Ca, CO_2 levels).

CBC AND BLOOD CULTURE

Order these as further follow-up tests, as indicated.

These test for sepsis and DIC.

OTHER TESTS

If the diagnosis remains unclear, consider the following:

- CSF tests: culture, protein, cytology, and glucose
- cardiac markers (troponin)

HEADACHE

KEYS TO WORKUP

Most cases of headache do not require laboratory testing. Lab testing is indicated if temporal arteritis or CNS infection is suspected.

LAB INVESTIGATIONS

LUMBAR PUNCTURE

Use this if you suspect CNS infection.

CRP OR ESR

Order a C-reactive protein (CRP) or an erythrocyte sedimentation rate (ESR) test if you suspect temporal arteritis.

MOVEMENT DISORDERS (BRADYKINETIC, HYPERKINETIC, OR TREMOR)

KEYS TO WORKUP

Bradykinetic movements are most often secondary to:

- drug-induced parkinsonism (e.g., neuroleptics, haloperidol, metoclopramide, verapamil, amiodarone, and prochlorperazine)

Hyperkinetic movement disorders include:

- myoclonus secondary to toxic or drug reaction
- metabolic disorders
- infection
- primary CNS conditions such as Parkinson, Huntington, and Alzheimer disease, and stroke

Tremors can occur secondarily to:

- Wilson disease
- medications (including amiodarone, lithium, and valproate)
- vitamin E deficiency

A complete history and physical examination, including drug history, may point toward a specific etiology and should direct laboratory testing.

LAB INVESTIGATIONS

Depending on patient history, testing may include:

- serum ceruloplasmin, and serum and urine copper levels with liver enzyme testing, for Wilson disease
- comprehensive urine drug screen and therapeutic drug monitoring
- vitamin E levels
- CSF analysis (culture, proteins, cytology, and glucose)
- metabolic screen (urine and serum electrolytes, blood gases, bicarbonate, and CO_2 levels)

SEIZURES

KEYS TO WORKUP

Primary unprovoked recurring seizures are designated as epileptic seizure disorders only after secondary causes have been excluded.

Secondary organic causes of seizure include:

- infection (febrile)
- metabolic causes such as hypo- or hyperglycemia, hypocalcemia, hyponatremia, uremia, and liver dysfunction

Other causes include eclampsia in pregnant women, drug overdose, and alcohol withdrawal.

Laboratory investigations can help rule out:

- drug ingestion and drug withdrawal
- infectious or febrile causes
- metabolic causes

LAB INVESTIGATIONS

TESTS FOR DRUG INGESTION AND DRUG WITHDRAWAL

Order the following tests as clinically indicated:

- serum alcohol
- urine drug screen

Note that if clinical findings are specific for a toxidrome, specify the suspected drugs or chemical substance.

See: intoxication and toxidromes, p. 173

TESTS FOR INFECTIOUS OR FEBRILE CAUSES

Order the following panel of investigations as clinically indicated:

- blood culture (to rule out bacterial meningitis or encephalitis)
- CBC (for cell and platelet counts to assess the risk of CNS thrombus or hemorrhage, and assess for evidence of exposure to toxins such as heavy metals)
- CSF (for culture, protein, cytology, and glucose to rule out autoimmune disease, bacterial or viral infection, and malignancy)
- peripheral smear (for morphological assessment of cells if CBC is abnormal, which is helpful in the diagnosis of underlying pathology)

TESTS FOR METABOLIC CAUSES

Order the following panel of investigations as clinically indicated:

- ABG (to assess anion gap, pH, bicarbonate, and CO_2 levels, which can affect electrolyte levels)
- creatinine/eGFR
- liver function tests: ALP, ALT, GGT (and, as indicated, AST, direct and indirect bilirubin, PT/INR)

LAB LITERACY FOR CANADIAN DOCTORS   225

- serum electrolytes
- urinalysis and urine protein

SYNCOPE

KEYS TO WORKUP

Causes of syncope are divided into benign and dangerous etiologies (see Table 26). Judicious use of lab testing may help differentiate some of these conditions in the appropriate clinical context.

However, the etiology of syncope is frequently undiagnosed even after extensive investigations. In 50% to 80% of patients, only a probable diagnosis is possible, since many cases are multifactorial.

Routine, unguided laboratory investigations are not recommended. Patient history and physical exam should guide any testing.

Table 26. Causes of syncope

Benign	Dangerous
Reflex-mediated (neurally mediated)	Cardiac arrhythmias or ischemia
Vasovagal	Transient ischemic attack (TIA)
Situational	Subarachnoid hemorrhage
Carotid sinus hypersensitivity	Subclavian steal migraines
Orthostatic causes (autonomic failure)	
Medications	
Postprandial hypotension	
Intravascular volume loss	

LAB INVESTIGATIONS

CARDIAC MARKERS (TROPONIN)

Order tests for troponin as clinically indicated. This is useful only if the patient history, physical exam, and ECG indicate concern for a cardiac cause.

CBC
Order this test if you suspect anemia.

See: anemia, p. 134

CREATININE AND ELECTROLYTES
Order these tests if confirmation of hydration status is required.

β-hCG
Order this for all women of childbearing age to rule out pregnancy, including ectopic pregnancy.

WEAKNESS AND SENSORY LOSS

KEYS TO WORKUP
A complete history and physical exam may point toward a specific etiology and direct decisions about testing.

Weakness and sensory loss can have multiple causes including:

- primary neuropathic and myopathic conditions (determined on physical exam, biopsy, and imaging)
- secondary causes (some detectable by laboratory testing)

Secondary causes detectable by laboratory testing include:

- myasthenia gravis
- botulism toxin
- anemia
- diabetes
- statin toxicity
- lead toxicity
- infection

LAB INVESTIGATIONS

COMPREHENSIVE URINE DRUG SCREEN

Order this test as clinically indicated to assess for weakness related to antiretroviral drugs, fibrates, neuromuscular blockers, statins, and steroids.

CBC AND PERIPHERAL BLOOD SMEAR

Order these tests as clinically indicated to assess for anemia and evidence of lead toxicity.

GLUCOSE MONITORING

Order the following tests as clinically indicated to rule out diabetes:

- fasting blood glucose
- HbA_{1c}

AChR ANTIBODY AND CLINICAL TENSILON TESTING

As clinically indicated, rule out myasthenia gravis by testing for acetylcholine receptor antibody (AChR antibody) and with Tensilon testing.

AChR antibody testing has:

- 50% sensitivity when myasthenia gravis is confined to the eyes
- 80% sensitivity when myasthenia gravis is generalized

CSF

Order CSF tests (culture, cytology, glucose, and protein) as clinically indicated to rule out autoimmune disease, bacterial or viral infection, and malignancies.

CK

Order a creatine kinase (CK) test as clinically indicated to assess for statin-related rhabdomyolysis.

MUSCLE BIOPSY

Use this test as clinically indicated to investigate neurogenic versus myogenic causes of weakness. Muscle and nerve fibre patterns on biopsy can distinguish between primary muscular disease (dystrophies) and primary neurologic disease (denervation, demyelination) along with inflammatory and storage disorders.

SEROLOGY

Use serology as clinically indicated to help rule out infectious and autoimmune causes of neuromuscular weakness.

WEIGHT LOSS OR GAIN

KEYS TO WORKUP

Weight loss and weight gain can be related to 3 major causes:

- increased or decreased caloric intake
- increased or decreased caloric expenditure
- secondary causes, which can include endocrine diseases, medications, and decreased mobility related to underlying medical conditions

Diseases associated with weight changes include:

- hypothyroidism
- adrenal dysfunction
- polycystic ovary syndrome
- hypogonadism
- congestive heart failure
- conditions that limit mobility

A number of medications may also be associated with changes in weight:

- antidiabetic medications (e.g., insulin, sulfonylureas, thiazolidinediones)
- antihypertensives (e.g., atenolol, metoprolol)

- corticosteroids (e.g., prednisone)
- antipsychotics (e.g., olanzapine, lithium), which increase appetite
- antidepressants (e.g., TCAs such as chlorpromazine and thioridazine; SSRIs such as paroxetine and fluoxetine)
- antihistamines, which cause lethargy
- anorexia medications, including amphetamine medications, antibiotics, antineoplastics, and bronchodilators

If clinical findings do not point to a likely cause, lab investigations can rule out some secondary causes.

- Start by ruling out hypothyroidism.
- Next, consider testing for adrenal dysfunction and other organic disease, which limit mobility or metabolism.

LAB INVESTIGATIONS

TESTS FOR HYPOTHYROIDISM

To follow up nonspecific clinical findings, begin by ruling out hypothyroidism.

- Start with TSH, which is the single best initial test for thyroid disorders.
- Follow up with a repeat TSH plus a T_4 if the initial TSH is elevated.

See: hypothyroidism, p. 37

TESTS FOR ORGANIC DISEASE

Consider the following tests if TSH rules out hypothyroidism:

- cortisol levels, dexamethasone suppression test for adrenal function (*see: adrenal disorders, p. 24*)
- CRP for other systemic inflammatory and chronic diseases

FURTHER READING

Ouyang H, Quinn J. Diagnosis and evaluation of syncope in the emergency department. *Emerg Med Clin North Am.* 2010;28(3):471–485. http://dx.doi.org/10.1016/j.emc.2010.03.007. Medline:20709239

Pereira AF, Simões do Couto F, de Mendonça A. The use of laboratory tests in patients with mild cognitive impairment. *J Alzheimers Dis.* 2006;10(1):53–58. Medline:16988482

Routine screening

Dr. Christopher Naugler

OVERALL APPROACH

The information in this section applies to asymptomatic patients on routine visits. It does not apply to symptomatic patients or patients with established disease, and the investigations they may require.

As much as possible, the information comes from published Canadian guidelines, or from an amalgamation of provincial guidelines where national guidelines do not exist.

Note that most screening guidelines recommend patient risk stratification as a first step. This limits screening to high-risk individuals and minimizes the harms associated with false-positive results.

COMMONLY ORDERED SCREENS

CA 125
Testing for cancer antigen 125 (CA 125) as way to screen for ovarian carcinoma is not recommended for the general population.

CBC
Screening via complete blood count (CBC) is not recommended for the general population.

CEA
Testing for carcinoembryonic antigen (CEA) as a way to screen for colorectal carcinoma is not recommended for the general population.

hsCRP
The only individuals recommended for high sensitivity C-reactive protein (hsCRP) screening are males older than 50, and females older than 60, with a low-density lipoprotein C (LDL-C) fraction less than 3.5 mmol/L (135 mg/dL). In these people, a hsCRP higher than 19.0 nmol/L (2.0 mg/L) may identify individuals who would benefit from statin therapy.

DIABETES

KEYS TO SCREENING

Screening for type 1 diabetes is not recommended for the general population.

All individuals should have their diabetes risk calculated (see Table 27). Screening for type 2 diabetes is recommended only for individuals at high risk.

PREFERRED SCREENING TESTS

HbA_{1c} (preferred)

Fasting plasma glucose

Oral glucose tolerance

FREQUENCY OF TESTING

Low- and moderate-risk patients: screening is not recommended.

High-risk patients: screen every 3 to 5 years.

Very high-risk patients: screen yearly.

PEARLS

HbA_{1c} testing to monitor known diabetics should not be performed more often than once every 3 months.

Table 27. FINDRISC diabetes risk stratification tool

Step 1: Calculate patient's total risk score		
Questions	Answer categories	Score
How old is your patient?	18–44	0 points
	45–54	2 points
	55–64	3 points
	65+	4 points

Continued on p. 234

Continued from p. 233

Questions	Answer categories	Score
What is your patient's body-mass index (BMI) or BMI category? See: Table 28	Normal (lower than 25.0 kg/m²)	0 points
	Overweight (25.0–29.9 kg/m²)	1 points
	Obese (30.0 kg/m² or higher)	3 points
What is your patient's waist circumference? Measure waist circumference below the ribs, usually at the level of the navel.	Men	
	< 94 cm (< ~37 in)	0 points
	94–102 cm (~37–40 in)	3 points
	> 102 cm (> ~40 in)	4 points
	Women	
	< 80 cm (< ~31 in)	0 points
	80–88 cm (~31–35 in)	3 points
	> 88 cm (> ~35 in)	4 points
Is your patient physically active for more than 30 minutes per day? Include physical activity during leisure, work, and regular daily routine.	Yes	0 points
	No	2 points
How often does your patient eat fruit and vegetables?	Every day	0 points
	Not every day	1 point
Has your patient ever taken medication for high blood pressure on a regular basis?	No	0 points
	Yes	2 points
Has your patient ever been found to have high blood glucose (e.g., in a health examination, during an illness, during pregnancy)?	No	0 points
	Yes	5 points
Do any members of the patient's family have type 1 or type 2 diabetes? Only count blood relatives.	No	0 points
	Yes: grandparent, aunt, uncle, first cousin (but no own parent, sibling, or child)	3 points
	Yes: parent, brother, sister, own child	5 points
		Total risk score: ____

Continued on p. 235

Continued from p. 234

Step 2: Match total risk score to degree of risk		
Score	**Risk category**	**Recommendations**
0–14 points	Low to moderate	Do not screen for type 2 diabetes
15–20 points	High risk	Screen every 3–5 years
21+ points	Very high risk	Screen every year

Reproduced by permission from the Canadian Task Force on Preventive Health Care.

Table 28. BMI chart

HEIGHT		BMI index or BMI range		
		Normal	**Overweight**	**Obese**
		(19.0–24.9 kg/m²)	**(25.0–29.9 kg/m²)**	**(30.0–39.0 kg/m²)**
m	**ft in**	**WEIGHT**		
1.47	4'10"	41–53 kg (91–117 lb)	54–64 kg (118–141 lb)	65–86 kg (142–189 lb)
1.50	4'11"	43–55 kg (94–122 lb)	56–66 kg (123–146 lb)	67–89 kg (147–196 lb)
1.52	5'0"	44–57 kg (97–126 lb)	58–68 kg (127–151 lb)	69–92 kg (152–202 lb)
1.55	5'1"	45–59 kg (100–130 lb)	59–71 kg (131–156 lb)	71–95 kg (157–209 lb)
1.57	5'2"	47–61 kg (104–134 lb)	62–73 kg (135–161 lb)	74–98 kg (162–216 lb)
1.60	5'3"	49–63 kg (107–138 lb)	63–75 kg (139–166 lb)	76–101 kg (167–223 lb)
1.63	5'4"	50–65 kg (110–143 lb)	66–78 kg (144–172 lb)	79–104 kg (173–230 lb)
1.65	5'5"	52–67 kg (114–147 lb)	68–80 kg (148–177 lb)	81–108 kg (178–237 lb)
1.68	5'6"	54–69 kg (118–151 lb)	70–83 kg (152–183 lb)	84–111 kg (184–244 lb)
1.70	5'7"	55–71 kg (121–156 lb)	71–85 kg (157–188 lb)	86–114 kg (189–252 lb)

Continued on p. 236

Continued from p. 235

HEIGHT		BMI index or BMI range		
		Normal	**Overweight**	**Obese**
		(19.0–24.9 kg/m²)	(25.0–29.9 kg/m²)	(30.0–39.0 kg/m²)
m	**ft in**	**WEIGHT**		
1.73	5'8"	57–73 kg (125–161 lb)	74–88 kg (162–194 lb)	88–117 kg (195–259 lb)
1.75	5'9"	58–75 kg (128–166 lb)	76–91 kg (167–200 lb)	92–121 kg (201–267 lb)
1.78	5'10"	60–78 kg (132–171 lb)	79–93 kg (172–206 lb)	94–125 kg (207–275 lb)
1.80	5'11"	62–80 kg (136–176 lb)	81–96 kg (177–212 lb)	97–128 kg (213–283 lb)
1.83	6'0"	64–82 kg (140–181 lb)	83–98 kg (182–217 lb)	99–132 kg (218–291 lb)
1.85	6'1"	65–84 kg (144–186 lb)	85–101 kg (187–223 lb)	102–136 kg (224–299 lb)
1.88	6'2"	67–86 kg (148–191 lb)	87–104 kg (191–229 lb)	105–139 kg (230–307 lb)
1.91	6'3"	69–89 kg (152–196 lb)	90–107 kg (197–236 lb)	108–143 kg (237–315 lb)
1.93	6'4"	71–91 kg (156–201 lb)	92–110 kg (202–242 lb)	111–147 kg (243–324 lb)

Reproduced by permission from the Canadian Task Force on Preventive Health Care.

See also: diabetes, p. 27

DYSLIPIDEMIA

KEYS TO SCREENING

Base your initial decision on whether to screen patients for dyslipidemia based on: sex, age, ethnic background, smoking history, and underlying medical conditions.

If you decide to screen, use the data from the initial tests to generate a Framingham risk score (see Table 29), which identifies patients at higher risk of developing cardiovascular disease within 10 years. This risk score should guide further decisions on treatment and frequency of testing.

Screening is generally recommended for:

- men older than 40
- women older than 50 or postmenopausal

Consider screening people at a younger age if they are descended from ethnic groups at a higher risk of developing dyslipidemia (South Asian, First Nations, and North American aboriginal populations).

Also consider screening smokers.

Medical conditions that may indicate a need to screen for dyslipidemia include:

- diabetes
- hypertension
- chronic renal disease
- obesity
- chronic obstructive pulmonary disease (COPD)
- systemic inflammatory disease
- HIV infection
- family history of premature cardiovascular disease or hyperlipidemia

Table 29. Framingham risk score: estimation of 10-year cardiovascular disease risk

Step 1: Calculate patient's total risk score		
	Risk points	
Risk factor	Men	Women
Age		
30–34	0	0
35–39	2	2
40–44	5	4

Continued on p. 238

Continued from p. 237

Risk factor	Risk points	
	Men	**Women**
Age		
45–49	6	5
50–54	8	7
55–59	10	8
60–64	11	9
65–69	12	10
70–74	14	11
75+	15	12
HDL-C		
≥ 1.6 mmol/L (≥ 60 mg/dL)	−2	−2
1.3–1.6 mmol/L (50–59 mg/dL)	−1	−1
1.2–1.3 mmol/L (45–49 mg/dL)	0	0
0.9–1.2 mmol/L (35–44 mg/dL)	1	1
< 0.9 mmol/L (< 35 mg/dL)	2	2
Total cholesterol		
< 4.1 mmol/L (< 160 mg/dL)	0	0
4.1–5.2 mmol/L (160–199 mg/dL)	1	1
5.2–6.2 mmol/L (200–239 mg/dL)	2	3
6.2–7.2 mmol/L (240–279 mg/dL)	3	4
≥ 7.2 mmol/L (≥ 280 mg/dL)	4	5

Continued on p. 239

Continued from p. 238

Risk factor	Risk points			
	Men		Women	
Systolic blood pressure (mmHg)	Not treated	Treated	Not treated	Treated
< 120	−2	0	−3	−1
120–129	0	2	0	2
130–139	1	3	1	3
140–149	2	4	2	5
150–159	2	4	4	6
160+	3	5	5	7
Diabetes				
Yes	3		4	
No	0		0	
Smoker				
Yes	4		3	
No	0		0	
Total points				

Step 2: Match total risk points to 10-year CVD risk (%)		
	10-year CVD risk (%)	
Total points	Men	Women
−3 or less	< 1	< 1
−2	1.1	< 1
−1	1.4	1.0
0	1.6	1.2
1	1.9	1.5
2	2.3	1.7

Continued on p. 240

Continued from p. 239

Total points	10-year CVD risk (%)	
	Men	Women
3	2.8	2.0
4	3.3	2.4
5	3.9	2.8
6	4.7	3.3
7	5.6	3.9
8	6.7	4.5
9	7.9	5.3
10	9.4	6.3
11	11.2	7.3
12	13.3	8.6
13	15.6	10.0
14	18.4	11.7
15	21.6	13.7
16	25.3	15.9
17	29.4	18.5
18	> 30	21.5
19	> 30	24.8
20	> 30	27.5
21+	> 30	> 30

Step 3: For patients between 30 and 59 years, double the CVD risk percentage if the patient has:

- a first-degree male relative who developed cardiovascular disease before age 55
- a first-degree female relative who developed cardiovascular disease before age 65

Reproduced by permission from *Circulation*.

PREFERRED SCREENING TEST

Lipid panel: total cholesterol, low-density lipoprotein cholesterol (LDL-C), high-density lipoprotein cholesterol (HDL-C), triglycerides

Note that:

- Increasingly, non-HDL-C and apolipoprotein B (APO-B) are being used as alternative lipid assessment targets, but availability and reporting may vary by laboratory.
- The following tests are recommended before beginning treatment with a statin:
  - ALT, creatinine/eGFR: renal dysfunction increases the risk of adverse effects of statins
  - creatine kinase (CK)
  - thyroid-stimulating hormone (TSH): hypothyroidism is a risk factor for statin-associated myopathy
  - urine protein: nephrotic syndrome may cause secondary dyslipidemia

FREQUENCY OF TESTING

Framingham risk score less than 5%: screen every 3 to 5 years.

Framingham risk score greater than or equal to 5%: screen yearly.

PEARLS

Total cholesterol and HDL cholesterol vary little with fasting: most individuals do not need to fast for these tests.

Exceptions are:

- individuals for whom triglycerides are the target of testing or treatment
- individuals being closely followed for LDL fraction (since LDL is calculated based on triglyceride level)

Note that:

- Non-HDL cholesterol is an alternative test, calculated from the standard lipid panel, and does not require fasting.

- APO-B is an alternative test to the lipid panel and also does not require fasting.

FECAL OCCULT BLOOD

KEYS TO SCREENING

Screening for fecal occult blood is based on individual risk of colorectal carcinoma.

Low-risk individuals are:

- younger than 50
- without a personal or family history of colon cancer, inflammatory bowel disease, or adenomatous polyps

Average-risk individuals are:

- otherwise at low risk, but 50 years of age or older

Moderate-risk individuals have at least 1 of the following factors:

- a personal history of colorectal carcinoma or adenomatous polyps
- a first-degree relative who developed colon cancer younger than 60
- at least 2 first-degree relatives diagnosed at any age

These guidelines refer only to asymptomatic individuals and do not refer to individuals with possible symptoms of colorectal carcinoma such as rectal bleeding.

PREFERRED SCREENING TESTS

Two tests are available for fecal occult blood: fecal immunochemical test (FIT) and guaiac fecal occult blood test (gFOBT, being phased out).

Note that:

- False positives and negatives may occur with either test, but particularly with gFOBT.

- gFOBT has a faster turnaround time than FIT, but has the following limitations:
  - ° gFOBT has false-negative results with vitamin C supplements, and false-positive results with certain foods.
  - ° In contrast to FIT, which is an automated test, gFOBT is a visual read: technologists can face challenges in distinguishing positive and negative results.
- FIT is more sensitive (and superior) to gFOBT: it detects as little as 0.3 mL of daily blood loss (as opposed to 10 mL for gFOBT).

FREQUENCY OF TESTING
Note that recommendations may vary by region: consult local colorectal carcinoma screening guidelines.

Low-risk individuals: screening is not recommended.

Average-risk individuals:

- Screen with FIT or gFOBT every 1 to 2 years from age 50 to 74.
- If a test is positive, refer the patient for colonoscopy.

Moderate-risk and high-risk individuals: screening with colonoscopy is recommended as per local guidelines.

PEARLS
A single gFOBT has a relatively low sensitivity (up to 30%), but 3 consecutive gFOBTs, or 2 consecutive FITs, have a sensitivity of 80%; the specificity is 98% to 99%.

PAP TEST

KEYS TO SCREENING
Screening is recommended for women between the ages of 25 and 69.

These recommendations apply to asymptomatic women, not those with symptoms of possible cancer (e.g., vaginal bleeding).

PREFERRED SCREENING TEST
Papanicolaou (Pap) test

FREQUENCY OF TESTING
Under age 25: do not screen.

Age 25–69: screen once every 3 years.

Over age 69: stop screening if patients have had 3 successive negative tests in the previous 10 years.

Note that abnormal results on a Pap test may necessitate increased frequency of testing. Check local guidelines.

PEARLS
There is inadequate evidence to make recommendations regarding HPV testing.

PSA

KEYS TO SCREENING
Base decisions about screening for prostate-specific antigen (PSA) on age and risk.

Consider using the following to evaluate risk:

- age-specific cut-offs (see Table 30)
- alternative measurements such as PSA velocity; a change in PSA velocity of more than 20% per year should prompt a referral for prostate biopsy

Higher-risk individuals may include:

- those with a first-degree relative diagnosed before age 65
- individuals of African descent

The age at which to begin screening in higher-risk individuals is not well established.

Note that:

- A digital rectal exam (DRE) provides useful information in addition to PSA.
- PSA should not be measured in patients with known active infection (e.g., urinary tract infection, prostatitis).

Table 30. Suggested PSA cut-off levels

Age	PSA value (ng/mL): general population	PSA value (ng/mL): individuals of African descent
40–49	2.5	2.0
50–59	3.5	4.0
60–69	4.5	4.5
70–79	6.5	5.5

PREFERRED SCREENING TEST
PSA

FREQUENCY OF TESTING
Men over age 50: after discussing the benefits and limitations of testing, screen yearly.

Men at higher risk of prostate cancer: after discussing the benefits and limitations of testing, screen yearly.

PEARLS
A number of consensus documents have suggested that any amount of PSA screening is harmful. This opinion stems primarily from the morbidity associated with surgical treatment of men with low-risk prostate carcinoma. Research on how to better manage these low-risk carcinomas may decrease the harms associated with testing.

SEXUALLY TRANSMITTED DISEASES
Indiscriminate screening for sexually transmitted diseases (STDs) is not recommended.

Base decisions to test for STDs on patient history, physical examination, and risk factors (e.g., individuals with a history of multiple sexual partners, sex workers and their clients, men who have sex with men).

Note that the incidence of specific infections varies regionally: refer to local guidelines.

THYROID FUNCTION

KEYS TO SCREENING

Screening is not recommended for the general population.

Testing is recommended for patients with both of the following:

- risk factors for thyroid disease
- signs and symptoms of thyroid disease

Risk factors for thyroid disease include:

- family history of thyroid disease, or personal history of thyroid or other autoimmune disease
- prior neck irradiation
- female and older than 50
- postpartum state (female): 6 weeks to 6 months
- male and elderly
- receiving lithium or amiodarone treatment

Signs and symptoms of thyroid disease include:

- weight gain or loss
- cold or heat intolerance
- menstrual changes
- constipation
- weakness
- tachycardia
- cognitive changes

PREFERRED SCREENING TEST

Thyroid-stimulating hormone (TSH)

Note that:

- A normal TSH should not be retested unless the clinical situation changes.
- An abnormal TSH (elevated signals hypothyroidism, suppressed signals hyperthyroidism) can be followed up with a free T_4 to confirm a diagnosis (*see: thyroid disorders, p. 33*).

FREQUENCY OF TESTING

Patients on a stable dose of thyroid medication: test yearly.

Patients with treated subclinical hypothyroidism: test yearly.

Following a thyroid medication dose adjustment, wait 8 to 12 weeks before testing.

ACUTE ILLNESS AND TSH

Avoid measuring TSH during a period of acute illness: euthyroid sick syndrome may result in thyroid function abnormalities that do not respond to thyroxine replacement. If TSH is measured in these patients, interpret the results with caution.

SUBCLINICAL HYPOTHYROIDISM

Subclinical hypothyroidism exists when:

- TSH is elevated but still below 10 mIU/L.
- Free T_4 is in the normal range.

Treatment is warranted in pregnancy and the presence of elevated thyroid peroxidase antibodies. Otherwise yearly testing of TSH should be performed.

T_3 TESTING: RARE

Free T_3 is used in the rare instance of suspected hyperthyroidism with a decreased TSH but a normal free T_4. In these cases, an elevated free T_3 confirms the diagnosis of hyperthyroidism.

See: hyperthyroidism, p. 33

VITAMIN B$_{12}$

KEYS TO SCREENING
Screening is not recommended for the general population.

Consider vitamin B_{12} testing in patients with:

- inflammatory small bowel disease
- gastric or small intestine resection
- prolonged vegan diet
- long-term use of H_2 receptor antagonists, proton pump inhibitors, or metformin
- malabsorption syndromes

Depending on the clinical presentation, consider testing for certain high-risk patients including:

- malnourished elderly patients
- institutionalized patients

PREFERRED SCREENING TEST
Vitamin B_{12}

FREQUENCY OF TESTING
This is not well established. A normal B_{12} level should not require retesting unless the clinical presentation changes.

PEARLS
Vitamin B_{12} testing has little role to play in the diagnosis of dementia and cognitive impairment. Vitamin B_{12} deficiency commonly occurs without macrocytic anemia, unless the degree of deficiency is severe.

VITAMIN D

KEYS TO SCREENING

Screening is not recommended for the general population.

Note that most individuals benefit from vitamin D supplementation, but testing is not medically necessary prior to or after starting supplements.

Testing may be indicated in certain high-risk populations, including those with:

- significant renal or liver disease
- malabsorption syndromes
- osteomalacia or osteoporosis

PREFERRED SCREENING TEST

25-hydroxyvitamin D

FREQUENCY OF TESTING

Allow at minimum a 4-month interval following dose supplement adjustment.

PEARLS

Vitamin D is one of the most misused of screening tests. A practice of "treating not testing" is appropriate for most individuals.

Therapeutic drug monitoring

Dr. Davinder Sidhu

ABBREVIATIONS

ASA	acetylsalicylic acid	PK	pharmacokinetics
AV	atrioventricular	PT	prothrombin time
CNS	central nervous system	PTT	partial thromboplastin time
DNA	deoxyribonucleic acid	SIADH	syndrome of inappropriate antidiuretic hormone secretion
GI	gastrointestinal		
NSAID	nonsteroidal anti-inflammatory drug	TDM	therapeutic drug monitoring

Principles of TDM

Therapeutic drug monitoring (TDM) is the measurement of serum drug levels to:

- assess for toxicity, overdose, and poisoning
- adjust dosages to achieve optimum clinical benefit

The 3 tables in this section give information relevant to both these objectives:

- Table 31 lists common drug classes that require TDM.

- Table 32 lists common medications monitored for therapeutic dosing and their reference ranges.
- Table 33 describes common clinical presentations associated with monitored drugs.

TDM FOR TOXICITY, OVERDOSE, AND POISONING

Consider TDM whenever a drug's therapeutic serum-concentration range approaches or overlaps its toxic serum-concentration range.

TDM FOR DOSE ADJUSTMENT

To use TDM effectively for dose adjustment, you need to understand basic pharmacokinetics (PK).

The first rule of PK is that serum levels must relate to therapeutic responses—otherwise TDM has no point. PK factors determine the relationship between dose and serum levels (see the breakdown that follows).

PK factor	Key concepts
Absorption	Factors that affect absorption include: • concurrent food intake • gastrointestinal (GI) metabolism • intestinal motility • malabsorption • variable expression of GI transporters
Bioavailability	Drugs usually bind to protein Factors that affect the circulating fraction bound include: • albumin levels • formulation (enteric coated pills) • solubility • stability Note that only the free drug is therapeutic and toxicologically active

Continued on p. 253

Continued from p. 252

PK factor	Key concepts
Compliance	This can be a major problem causing subtherapeutic drug levels, particularly in psychiatric or elderly patients with memory issues
Metabolism	After a drug is absorbed, it is either metabolized or eliminated
	Metabolic breakdown may activate or deactivate the drug due to:
	• interactions between the drug and metabolites
	• limited availability of key substances required for key metabolic pathways
Renal disease or liver disease	These conditions may clear many drugs unmetabolized
Volume of distribution	Drug size and solubility affect distribution
	Extremely hydrophilic (lipophobic) drugs stay in vascular space
	Hydrophobic (lipophilic) drugs penetrate extravascular space and adipose tissue

When dosing a patient with a medication, your goal is optimal therapeutic response with minimum risk of toxic side effects.

If the dosage required is variable, but the drug has a narrow therapeutic range, work from the following principles:

- Start with a small dose and increase the dose until the desired effect is seen.
- Drugs are dosed according to half-life (the time it takes for the serum concentration of a drug to reach half its starting amount): if a drug's half-life is 12 hours, then dosing is usually every 12 hours to maintain therapeutic levels.

BLOOD DRAWS FOR TDM

For valid results, blood samples must meet both these criteria:

- taken at the appropriate time
- taken after the administration of a sufficient number of doses

Some drugs, especially antibiotics, require draws for peak and trough levels:

- peak levels: draw at the point of maximum drug absorption
- trough levels: draw just before the next dose

Most TDM testing is conducted through commercial immunoassay techniques, although some laboratories employ gas or liquid chromatography to test for drug analytes or metabolites.

TDM tables

Table 31. Common drug classes that require TDM

Drug class	Examples
Antiasthmatics	Theophylline
Antibiotics (aminoglycosides)	Gentamicin
	Tobramycin
	Vancomycin
Anticonvulsants	Carbamazepine
	Phenytoin
Cardiac antiarrhythmics and glycosides	Antiarrhythmics
	Lidocaine
	Procainamide
	Glycosides
	Digoxin
Lithium	Lithium compounds
Nonsteroidal anti-inflammatory drugs	Salicylate

Table 32. Reference ranges for common medications monitored for therapeutic dosing*

Drug	Therapeutic range	Toxic level
Acetaminophen**	70–130 µmol/L (5–20 µg/mL)	> 260 µmol/L (> 40 µg/mL)
Amikacin	peak: 34–51 µmol/L (20–30 µg/mL)	peak: > 60 µmol/L (> 35 µg/mL)
	trough: 7–14 µmol/L (4–8 µg/mL)	trough: > 17 µmol/L (> 10 µg/mL)
Amitriptyline	433–540 nmol/L (120–150 ng/mL)	> 805 nmol/L (> 500 ng/ml)
Carbamazepine	21–51 µmol/L (5–12 µg/mL)	> 51 µmol/L (> 12 µg/mL)
Clonazepam	40–200 nmol/L (15–60 ng/mL)	> 260 nmol/L (> 80 ng/mL)
Desipramine	563–1125 nmol/L (150–300 ng/mL)	> 1875 nmol/L (> 500 ng/mL)
Diazepam	1.75–7.0 nmol/L (0.5–2 mg/L)	> 11 nmol/L (> 3 mg/L)
Digoxin	1–2.6 nmol/L (0.8–2 ng/mL)	> 2.6 nmol/L (> 2 ng/mL)
Disopyramide	6–15 µmol/L (2–5 µg/mL)	> 21 µmol/L (> 7 µg/mL)
Ethosuximide	280–708 µmol/L (40–100 µg/mL)	> 1062 µmol/L (> 150 µg/mL)
Flecainide	0.5–2.4 µmol/L (0.2–1 µg/mL)	> 2.4 µmol/L (> 1 µg/mL)
Gentamicin	peak: 12–21 µmol/L (6–10 µg/mL)	peak: > 24 µmol/L (> 12 µg/mL)
	trough: < 4 µmol/L (< 2 µg/mL)	trough: > 4 µmol/L (> 2 µg/mL)
Imipramine	535–1070 nmol/L (150–300 ng/mL)	> 1785 nmol/L (> 500 ng/mL)
Lidocaine	6–21 µmol/L (1.5–5 µg/mL)	> 21 µmol/L (> 5 µg/mL)
Lithium	0.5–1.5 mmol/L (0.5–1.5 mEq/L)	> 1.5 mmol/L (> 1.5 mEq/L)
Nortriptyline	190–570 nmol/L (50–150 ng/mL)	> 1900 nmol/L (> 500 ng/mL)
Phenobarbital	66–132 µmol/L (15–30 µg/mL)	> 177 µmol/L (> 40 µg/mL)
Phenytoin	40–80 µmol/L (10–20 µg/mL)	> 80 µmol/L (> 20 µg/mL)
Primidone	23–55 µmol/L (5–12 µg/mL)	> 69 µmol/L (> 15 µg/mL)

Continued on p. 256

Continued from p. 255

Drug	Therapeutic range	Toxic level
Procainamide	17–42 µmol/L (4–10 µg/mL)	> 68 µmol/L (> 16 µg/mL)
Quinidine	6–15 µmol/L (2–5 µg/mL)	> 31 µmol/L (>10 µg/mL)
Salicylic acid**	0.7–1.8 mmol/L (100–250 µg/mL)	> 2.2 mmol/L (> 300 µg/mL)
Theophylline	55–111 µmol/L (10–20 µg/mL)	> 111 µmol/L (> 20 µg/mL)
Tobramycin	peak: 11–21 µmol/L (5–10 µg/mL) trough: < 4 µmol/L (< 2 µg/mL)	peak: > 26 µmol/L (> 12 µg/mL) trough: > 4 µmol/L (> 2 µg/mL)
Valproic acid	347–693 µmol/L (50–100 µg/mL)	> 693 µmol/L (> 100 µg/mL)
Vancomycin	peak: 14–28 µmol/L (20–40 µg/mL) trough: 7–14 µmol/L (10–20 µg/mL)	peak: > 55 µmol/L (> 80 µg/mL) trough: > 14 µmol/L (>20 µg/mL)

*These values are a general guide only and should not replace the reference ranges provided by the reporting laboratory.

**Although these are not routinely monitored as part of TDM, they have actionable toxic ranges.

Table 32. Reference ranges for common medications monitored for therapeutic dosing

Drug	Therapeutic range	Toxic level
Acetaminophen*	70–130 µmol/L (5–20 µg/mL)	> 130 µmol/L (> 40 µg/mL)
Amikacin	peak: 34–51 µmol/L (20–30 µg/mL) trough: 7–14 µmol/L (4–8 µg/mL)	peak: > 60 mol/L (> 35 µg/mL) trough: > 51 µmol/L (> 10 µg/mL)
Amitriptyline	433–903 nmol/L (120–150 ng/mL)	> 805 nmol/L (> 500 ng/ml)
Carbamazepine	21–51 µmol/L (5–12 µg/mL)	> 51 µmol/L (> 12 µg/mL)
Clonazepam	40–200 µmol/L (15–60 ng/mL)	> 260 nmol/L (> 80 ng/mL)
Desipramine	281–1125 nmol/L (150–300 ng/mL)	> 1500 nmol/L (> 500 ng/mL)
Diazepam	0.35–3.5 nmol/L (0.5–2 mg/L)	> 17.5 nmol/L (> 3 mg/L)
Digoxin	1–2.6 nmol/L (0.8–2 ng/mL)	> 2.6 nmol/L (> 2 ng/mL)
Disopyramide	9–18 µmol/L (2–5 µg/mL)	> 21 µmol/L (> 7 µg/mL)
Ethosuximide	280–708 µmol/L (40–100 µg/mL)	> 1062 µmol/L (> 150 µg/mL)
Flecainide	0.5–2.4 µmol/L (0.2–1 µg/mL)	> 2.4 µmol/L (> 1 µg/mL)
Gentamicin	peak: 12–21 µmol/L (6–10 µg/mL) trough: < 4 µmol/L (< 2 µg/mL)	peak: > 21 µmol/L (> 12 µg/mL) trough: > 4 µmol/L (> 2 µg/mL)
Imipramine	610–1670 nmol/L (150–300 ng/mL)	> 1785 nmol/L (> 500 ng/mL)
Lidocaine	6–21 µmol/L (1.5–5 µg/mL)	> 39 µmol/L (> 5 µg/mL)
Lithium	0.5–1.5 mmol/L (0.5–1.5 mEq/L)	> 1.5 mmol/L (> 1.5 mEq/L)
Nortriptyline	190–570 nmol/L (50–150 ng/mL)	> 1900 nmol/L (> 500 ng/mL)
Phenobarbitone	86–172 µmol/L (15–30 µg/mL)	> 172 µmol/L (> 40 µg/mL)
Phenytoin	40–80 µmol/L (10–20 µg/mL)	> 158 µmol/L (> 20 µg/mL)

Continued on p. 256

Continued from p. 255

Drug	Therapeutic range	Toxic level
Primidone	23–55 µmol/L (5–12 µg/mL)	> 55 µmol/L (> 12 µg/mL)
Procainamide	17–42 µmol/L (4–10 µg/mL)	> 51 µmol/L (> 10 µg/mL)
Quinidine	6–15 µmol/L (2–5 µg/mL)	> 29 µmol/L (> 6 µg/mL)
Salicylic acid*	1–2 mmol/L (10–30 mg/dL)	> 3.6 mmol/L (> 35 mg/dL)
Theophylline	28–111 µmol/L (10–20 µg/mL)	> 111 µmol/L (> 20 µg/mL)
Tobramycin	peak: 13–21 µmol/L (6–10 µg/mL)	peak: > 21 µmol/L (> 12 µg/mL)
	trough: < 4 µmol/L (< 2 µg/mL)	trough: > 4 µmol/L (> 2 µg/mL)
Valproic acid	350–700 µmol/L	> 1386 µmol/L
Vancomycin	peak: 14–28 µmol/L (20–40 µg/mL)	peak: > 28 µmol/L (> 80 µg/mL)
	trough: 3–7 µmol/L (5–10 µg/mL)	trough: > 21 µmol/L (> 10 µg/mL)

*Although these are not routinely monitored as part of TDM, they have actionable toxic ranges.

Table 33. Common clinical presentations associated with monitored therapeutic agents

Presentation	Drug/medication	Clinical pearls
Arrhythmia	Insulin • increases K$^+$ intracellular shifts Digoxin, beta-2 blocker (e.g., propranolol) • affect potassium channel function to prevent intracellular shift of K$^+$ in hyperkalemia Potassium-sparing diuretics • reduce potassium excretion	Insulin can cause a massive K$^+$ intracellular shift resulting in hypokalemia
	Quinidine, phenothiazines, and tricyclic antidepressants • cause prolonged QT (common) Loop diuretics and thiazide diuretics • increase renal excretion of potassium	Quinidine and amiodarone both affect free digoxin levels and impair clearance

Continued on p. 257

Continued from p. 256

Presentation	Drug/medication	Clinical pearls
Ataxia and falling	**Polypharmacy** • is especially a concern with > 4 medications in the elderly **Phenytoin** • causes prolonged PR due to AV block, horizontal gaze nystagmus, and incoordination **Quinidine** • toxic levels cause altered mental status, tinnitus, vertigo, blurred vision, and prolonged QT	
Bleeding/bruising	**Steroids** • cause vascular dysfunction **ASA** • causes disordered platelet function **Warfarin (Coumadin)** • vitamin K antagonist • prevents clotting by inhibiting activity of vitamin K–dependent coagulation factors **Heparin** • factor IIa (thrombin) inhibitor • prevents fibrin clot crosslinking • mechanism of action increases activity of factor III (antithrombin) negative feedback to limit thrombin levels	PT is more sensitive to vitamin K deficiency and is used to monitor Coumadin therapy PTT is more sensitive to heparin and is used to monitor therapy
Confusion and decreased levels of consciousness	**Thiazide diuretics and other drugs causing SIADH** • cause hyponatremia	
Constipation	**Opiates, antihypertensives, and Ca-channel blockers** • affect peristaltic gut motility **Anticholinergics (antispasmodics, antidepressants, anti-Parkinson, and antipsychotics)** **Iron** • affects gut flora	Anticholinergics decrease acetycholine stimulation through muscarinic receptor blockades

Continued on p. 258

Continued from p. 257

Presentation	Drug/medication	Clinical pearls
Drug-induced autoimmune disorders	Procainamide, hydralazine, and isoniazid • cause drug-induced lupus	The mechanism of causation is uncertain, but may involve induction of antihistone antibodies
Hepatomegaly	Alcohol, NSAIDs, amiodarone, methotrexate, chlorpromazine, erythromycin (and others) • cause alcohol- and drug-induced hepatitis, and fatty liver	Increased inflammation secondary to medication effect is often due to reduced or impaired hepatic metabolism from the drugs
Hypercalcemia	Excess vitamin D Thiazide diuretics Lithium Vitamin A/isotretinoin	Drug side effects are usually independent of PTH levels, unlike most other causes Excess vitamin D may also result in hyperphosphatemia due to increased absorption Thiazide diuretics and acetazolamide cause hypophosphatemia due to increased excretion
Hyperglycemia	Corticosteroids • stimulate gluconeogenesis in the liver Thiazide diuretics • are associated with increased risk of developing type 2 diabetes with chronic use Beta-agonists (e.g., Salbutamol) • stimulate hepatic glycogen breakdown (glycogenolysis) and pancreatic release of glucagon, which work together to increase plasma glucose	

Continued on p. 259

Continued from p. 258

Presentation	Drug/medication	Clinical pearls
Hypoglycemia	Insulin and insulin secretagogues Beta-adrenergic antagonists Quinidine Salicylate Pentamidine	Insulin and medications that increase insulin production may rapidly shift glucose intracellularly
Hypothyroidism, chronic	Thionamides Lithium Amiodarone Interferon	Amiodarone causes: • thyroid toxicity • hypothyroidism (5%–15%) • hyperthyroidism (1%-2%) • pulmonary toxicity (1%) • hepatic toxicity (0.6%)
Metabolic acidosis	Metformin, isoniazid • causes excess acids due to lactic acidosis Salicylate	Medications usually cause excess acid; unless nephrotoxic, they rarely affect acid excretion or bicarbonate production to cause acidosis
Metabolic alkalosis	Loop diuretics (e.g., Furosemide) and thiazide diuretics	Diuretics cause renal losses of sodium, which result in contraction alkalosis
Nausea and vomiting	Chemotherapy, alcohol, and antibiotics	
Neuropathy	Aminoglycosides (e.g., Gentamicin) • cause acoustic neuropathy Amiodarone • causes peripheral neuropathy	Gentamicin dosing must be based on renal function, which affects clearance
Renal dysfunction, acute or chronic	Lithium • is directly nephrotoxic for renal tubular cells	Lithium has a narrow therapeutic window and must be monitored at 1–3 month intervals for evidence of renal toxicity

Continued on p. 260

Presentation	Drug/medication	Clinical pearls
Respiratory acidosis (hypoventilation)	Opiates (e.g., morphine, fentanyl) Barbiturates (e.g., phenobarbital) Benzodiazepines (e.g., temazepam)	Most medications act through CNS respiratory depression mechanisms and often have a synergistic effect when combined
Respiratory alkalosis (hyperventilation)	Salicylate • causes direct respiratory center stimulation	Toxicity is characterized by hyperventilation resulting from direct respiratory centre stimulation, leading to respiratory alkalosis and compensatory alkaluria
Thrombocytopenia	Quinidine • causes immune-mediated platelet destruction Methotrexate • folate antagonist • decreases DNA production Chemotherapeutic agents (e.g., cisplatin, cytosine arabinoside, and vincristine) • cause toxic damage to bone marrow	Medications are typically implicated in decreased platelet production or increased immune-mediated peripheral destruction

FURTHER READING

Lab basics

Dr. Christopher Naugler

Interpreting abnormal results

Lab tests that deliver false-positive results, or abnormal but clinically insignificant results, can burden patients with unnecessary worry. They can also burden the health care system with unnecessary costs, especially since misleading results can lead to unnecessary follow-up tests.

WHY HEALTHY PATIENTS SOMETIMES HAVE ABNORMAL TEST RESULTS

Physicians are inundated with laboratory test results on a regular basis. Often, we have to make split-second decisions about what test results need follow-up action. Fortunately, laboratories make this easier by labelling results as normal or abnormal on their reports.

However, here's the problem with this helpful addition to patient test results: healthy patients can have abnormal test results. Why does this happen? To answer this we need to look at how laboratories determine what is "normal."

Laboratories take samples from "normal," healthy volunteers and create distribution graphs of the results. Most results cluster around some measure of central tendency (the mean or median), and a smaller number fall outside the central tendency (see Figure 14). By convention, the normal range for many test results is defined as the middle 95% of results for healthy individuals. Any results falling above or below this range are defined as abnormal, even though they are perfectly normal for about 5% of healthy people.

What this means in practice is that—on average, for any given test—5% of healthy people will have a result outside the normal range. So if you want to find an abnormal result on a healthy patient, all you need to do is order more tests! Figure 15 shows the problem this poses for interpreting laboratory test results: it plots the probability of finding an abnormal result as a function of how many tests are ordered. Remember that this is the probability of finding an

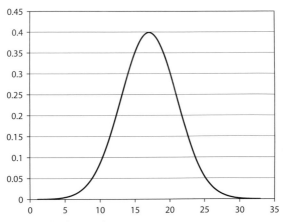

Figure 14. Distribution graph

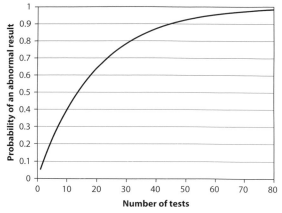

Figure 15. Probability of an abnormal result as number of lab tests rises

abnormal result in a *healthy* individual. As you can see, starting at about 12 tests, the chance of getting at least one abnormal result is higher than 50%.

HOW TO IDENTIFY FALSE OR CLINICALLY INSIGNIFICANT RESULTS

So, you might ask, how can I trust that any test result is not a false positive? The short answer is that you can never be certain, but you can make a sound assessment by using one of the most powerful reasoning tools available to every clinician: the differential diagnosis. Just like clinical presentations, laboratory test results have a differential diagnosis. This differential consists of several possibilities.

For an abnormal result:

1) The result is real (and may or may not be indicative of disease).
2) The result is a false positive (i.e., the result of testing error).

For a normal result:

1) The result is real (and may or may not indicate the absence of disease).
2) The result is a false negative (i.e., the result of a testing error).

The relative probability of which answer/diagnosis is correct depends on the pretest probabilities. Once you are in the mindset of considering a differential for a test result, this process becomes surprisingly easy:

- Was there a clinical presentation consistent with the result you obtained (i.e., a high pretest probability)? If yes, then the result is likely "real."
- Was this an "out of the blue" result on a healthy patient (especially a marginally abnormal result in a long series of tests)? If yes, then a normal value outside the normal range or a "false positive" is more likely. This is why clinicians are cautioned against conducting "screening" tests in low-risk individuals.

WHAT TO DO ABOUT UNEXPECTED ABNORMAL RESULTS

SEVERELY ABNORMAL RESULTS

Severely abnormal unexpected results should obviously be repeated immediately (or may need to be acted upon in emergency situations).

MARGINALLY ABNORMAL RESULTS

Depending on your level of clinical judgement, you may choose to ignore marginally abnormal results in clinically healthy individuals. You can also usually treat them with "tincture of time": false-positive results will tend to move toward a less extreme value on repeated testing. This is essentially a statistical phenomenon based on the fact that a given result for a patient is really a number drawn from a distribution of numbers representing the range of normal for that patient. Because extreme results are less commonly encountered (think of the tails of a bell curve), repeat testing will likely sample values from the centre of the distribution, therefore giving less extreme values—a phenomenon known as *regression to the mean*.

If you consider further testing necessary, a good strategy always is to repeat tests with abnormal results at a later point to see if they return to normal.

ABOUT NORMAL RANGE

You should also keep in mind that the normal range for a given test:

- is often different for adults and children
- may vary between males and females
- may vary among laboratories

The laboratory that performed the test is always the best source for the normal range and is also a good place to ask for help with test interpretation.

Lab errors

WHAT TO DO IF YOU SUSPECT A LAB ERROR

There are instances where a lab result is so at odds with the clinical presentation that error must enter into your differential diagnosis. In these cases, 2 things should happen:

- the patient should be retested (if possible)
- the reporting laboratory should be contacted and informed of your concerns

If there really was an error, other patients may have been affected. Blood samples are usually stored for several days before discarding, so, if you notify the laboratory quickly, the lab may be able to retest the specimen. Even if this is not possible, laboratories have a number of investigative tools at their disposal to help detect errors.

LAB ERRORS AND PHYSICIAN ERRORS

When we think of laboratory errors, we generally point to analytical errors by the laboratory itself. But most errors in testing occur before specimens reach the lab (preanalytic errors) or after the lab releases results (postanalytic errors).

Some errors, in other words, are under the control of clinicians.

When our own laboratory investigates presumed errors, the majority turn out to be preanalytic. Preanalytic errors include:

- wrong test ordered for the clinical presentation
- specimen from the wrong patient
- specimen inadequate for diagnosis
- specimen in the wrong container or tube (so, in the wrong additive or preservative)
- specimen destruction from environmental factors (e.g., freezing or overheating in transit)
- specimen never delivered to the laboratory or delivered after too much time had passed
- error in data entry for the specimen

Postanalytic errors include:

- misinterpretation of lab report by clinician
- report filed or discarded before clinician saw it

It is important for clinicians to be aware of these errors when they receive a test result that doesn't make sense. Moreover, an awareness of these possibilities allows clinicians to examine their own practices to identify potential processes vulnerable to these errors.

The key preventative actions are:

- Ensure that requisitions are completely filled out.
- Watch out for label transposition on specimens. Take special care if you collect blood from more than one patient or do more than one procedure (e.g., Pap test or biopsy) in a day.
- Deliver specimens to the lab in a timely fashion.
- Call your lab if you have questions about specimen types, test selection, or report interpretation.

Protocols for specimen collection

Proper protocols for specimen collection reduce preanalytic errors, and ensure the best use of time and money in laboratory testing.

ANATOMIC AND CYTOPATHOLOGY SPECIMENS

The guidelines given here are appropriate for inpatient or office-based procedures. Specialized procedures such as large surgical resections, lymphoma protocols, and bone marrow biopsies are beyond the scope of this book.

PROVIDE SPECIMENS PLUS CLINICAL FINDINGS

When you submit samples for interpretation by anatomic or general pathologists (histology) or cytopathologists (single cell morphology), provide details of the clinical history and presentation. Accurate interpretation of many specimens depends on the provision of an accurate clinical history.

WHEN IN DOUBT, CONSULT THE PATHOLOGIST

A wide array of diagnoses may arise from anatomic and histological evaluation. If in doubt of the significance of an interpretation or the appropriate management, a call to the reporting pathologist is often the easiest way to determine further management.

ABOUT BIOPSY SPECIMENS

Provide a generous amount of tissue, if possible. The smaller the tissue sample, the greater the possibility of false-negative results or misdiagnosis.

Take special care with small tissue samples. Small samples may stick to the side or cap of the container, and therefore not become properly fixed. This means the lab may not be able to analyze them.

- Make sure you can see the tissue in the formalin before you put the cap on the specimen jar.
- If a larger specimen appears to be floating, place a small piece of paper towel on the surface of the formalin to ensure that the specimen remains below the surface.

Use separate jars for specimens that come from different locations on the same patient. If you put them in the same jar, and one specimen is unexpectedly malignant, you may have great difficulty determining where the malignant specimen came from.

FIXED SPECIMENS

Fix all specimens for histological examination.

To fix, place the specimens immediately in a 10% formalin solution. Ensure at least a 10:1 ratio of formalin to volume of tissue. A 20:1 ratio is even better.

FRESH (UNFIXED) SPECIMENS

Always provide fresh, unfixed specimens from lymph node biopsies; notify the pathologist in advance when you are preforming a lymph node biopsy.

Note that microbiologic culture studies cannot be performed on fixed tissue specimens. Consider providing fresh specimens, in addition to fixed specimens, for:

- infectious dermatitis
- vesiculobullous dermatoses
- vasculitides

Submit fresh skin specimens moist in saline gauze.

BIOPSY PROCEDURES

Choose the right biopsy procedure for the type of specimen:

- excisional biopsy: required for pigmented skin lesions
- open biopsy: preferred for lymph nodes, because it allows evaluation of architecture, microorganisms, and abnormal cell populations
- punch biopsy: required for cutaneous processes with suspected involvement of the dermis, because it provides a representative sample of the epidermis and full-thickness dermis; larger punch biopsies also sample subcutaneous fat
- shave biopsy: suitable for skin conditions involving only the epidermis

ABOUT CYTOLOGY SPECIMENS

Methodologies for cytology vary considerably from laboratory to laboratory.

Some laboratories perform "conventional" cytology, where the sample is smeared on a glass slide and immediately sprayed with a tissue fixative.

Many cytology departments have switched to so-called liquid-based cytology, where samples are submitted to the lab in a proprietary media. In these instances you need to:

- obtain specimen submission containers from your lab
- confirm the proper procedure for sample collection

BLOOD

If you perform blood draws:

- Make sure you use the correct order of draw and collection tubes for blood specimens. Table 34 shows an example order of draw: always check protocols with the laboratory you use.
- Fill the tubes to the correct level: this ensures the correct ratio of additives to blood.
- Refrigerate samples promptly.
- Deliver them to the lab promptly. Samples for general chemistry testing (e.g., electrolytes, creatinine, glucose, etc.) need to be spun (the liquid and cellular elements separated) within 2 hours of collection, preferably sooner.

Table 34. Order of blood draw*

Order of draw	Colour of stopper	Invert	Additive	Comments
1	Clear	N/A	None	Tube used only as a discard tube
2	Blood culture bottle	Invert gently to mix	Bacterial growth medium and activated charcoal	When a culture is ordered along with any other blood work, the blood cultures **must** be drawn first
3	Yellow (with a clear label)	8–10 times	Sodium polyanethol sulfonate (SPS)	Tube used for mycobacteria (AFB) blood culture
4	Royal blue (with red band on label)	N/A	Glass tube with no additive	Tube used for copper and zinc

Continued on p. 271

Continued from p. 270

Order of draw	Colour of stopper	Invert	Additive	Comments
5	Red **glass**	N/A	Glass tube with no additive	Tube used for serum tests, which **cannot** be collected in SST tubes **Note:** red PLASTIC tubes are preferable for lab tests
6	Light blue	3–4 times	Sodium citrate anticoagulant	Tube used mainly for PT (INR), PTT, and other coagulation studies
7	Black **glass**	3–4 times	Sodium citrate anticoagulant	Tube used for ESR **only**
8	Red	5 times	Clot activator and no anticoagulant	Tube used for serum tests, which **cannot** be collected in SST tubes
9	Gold	5 times	Gel separator and clot activator	Usually referred to as "SST" (serum separator tube) After centrifugation, the gel forms a barrier between the clot and the serum
10	Dark green **glass** (with rubber stopper)	8–10 times	Glass tube with sodium heparin anticoagulant	Tube used for antimony
11	Dark green	8–10 times	Sodium heparin anticoagulant	Tube used mainly for amino acids and cytogenetics tests
12	Light green (mint)	8–10 times	Lithium heparin anticoagulant and gel separator	Usually referred to as "PST" (plasma separator tube) After centrifugation, the gel forms a barrier between the blood cells and the plasma Tube used mainly for chemistry tests

Continued on p. 272

Continued from p. 271

Order of draw	Colour of stopper	Invert	Additive	Comments
13	Royal blue (with blue band on label)	8–10 times	K_2EDTA anticoagulant	Tube used for trace elements
14	Royal blue (with lavender band on label)	8–10 times	Na_2EDTA anticoagulant	Tube used for lead
15	Lavender	8–10 times	EDTA anticoagulant	Tube used mainly for CBC, pretransfusion testing, hemoglobin A_1c, and antirejection drugs **Note:** EDTA tubes specifically for catecholamines also include sodium metabisulfite
16	Yellow (with yellow-banded white label)	8–10 times	Acid citrate dextrose solution "A" (ACDA)	Tube used for tissue typing and some flow cytometry testing
17	Grey	8–10 times	Sodium fluoride and potassium oxalate anticoagulant	Tube used for lactate

*These are the 2013 protocols of Calgary Laboratory Services.

Reproduced by permission from Calgary Laboratory Services.

Lab investigations index

Dr. Christopher Naugler and
Dr. Leland B. Baskin

This index describes the diagnostic purpose of the lab investigations discussed in this guide, plus other common lab tests.

Clinicians often work with patients who have already had lab tests done, and whose results require interpretation. This index provides a quick way to check key information.

Test	Specimen	Clinical utility
17-Hydroxyprogesterone	Blood	Detection of congenital adrenal hyperplasia
ABG (arterial blood gas)	Blood	Assessment of oxygen–carbon dioxide exchange
		Assessment of acid-base status
Acetaminophen	Blood	Assessment and management of acetaminophen overdose
Acetone	Blood	Elevated acetone levels indicate isopropyl alcohol ingestion
AChE (acetylcholinesterase)	Blood	Evaluation of pesticide exposure

Continued on p. 274

Continued from p. 273

Test	Specimen	Clinical utility
AChR antibody (acetylcholine receptor antibody)	Blood (chilled or frozen)	Diagnosis of myasthenia gravis: 85% of patients have this antibody
ACTH (adrenocorticotropic hormone)	Blood	Elevated ACTH levels point to Addison disease, congenital adrenal hyperplasia, and pituitary tumours producing ACTH Depressed levels point to Cushing disease and pituitary failure
Acute leukemia panel	Blood	Diagnosis of leukemia and lymphoma
ADH (antidiuretic hormone)	Blood	Elevated ADH levels may indicate syndrome of inappropriate antidiuretic hormone (SIADH)
	Urine	Depressed levels may indicate diabetes insipidus
AFP (α_1-fetoprotein)	Blood	Follow-up of patients with certain testicular and ovarian tumours, and hepatocellular carcinoma Prenatal screening Note: AFP is naturally elevated in neonates
AG (anion gap)	Blood	Assessment of acid-base disorders *See p. 292 for calculation and other details*
Albumin	Blood	Assessment of liver and kidney disease, and nutritional status
Albumin—urine (microalbumin)	24-hour urine collection	Diagnosis of renal disease
	Timed urine collection	Monitoring of chronic renal disease
	Random urine specimen	
ALC-1 (anti–liver cytosol antibody type 1)	Blood	Diagnosis of autoimmune hepatitis
Aldosterone	Blood	With renin, diagnosis of hyperaldosteronism

Continued on p. 275

Continued from p. 274

Test	Specimen	Clinical utility
Aldosterone—urine	24-hour urine collection	Assessment of adrenal disorders
ALKM-1 (anti–liver kidney microsomal antibody type 1)	Blood	Diagnosis of autoimmune hepatitis
Allergy testing, IgE	Blood	Diagnosis of IgE-mediated allergy Note: a negative specific IgE antibody test should not be used on its own to reject a diagnosis of allergy (it is possible for a patient to have significant allergy yet have a negative test)
ALP (alkaline phosphatase)	Blood	Elevated values point to liver disease and bone diseases Assessment of disease activity in Paget disease
ALT (alanine transaminase)	Blood	Assessment of liver disease and damage Note: ALT is a more specific marker than AST
Ammonia	Blood	Assessment of liver disease
Amylase	Blood	Diagnosis of pancreatitis
ANA (antinuclear antibody)	Blood	Diagnosis of numerous autoimmune diseases
ANCA (neutrophil cytoplasmic antibody)	Blood	Diagnosis of a number of autoimmune disorders
Anti-GBM (anti–glomerular basement membrane)	Blood	Elevated anti-GBM levels may indicate Goodpasture syndrome
Antiphospholipid antibody (cardiolipin antibody)	Blood	Diagnosis of antiphospholipid antibody syndrome
Anti-*Saccharomyces cerevisiae* antibody	Blood	Differentiating Crohn disease (usually positive) from ulcerative colitis (usually negative)
Antithrombin	Blood	Antithrombin deficiency is one cause of thrombophilia
Anti-TPO (anti–thyroid peroxidase)	Blood	Anti-TPO is often associated with Hashimoto thyroiditis

Continued on p. 276

Continued from p. 275

Test	Specimen	Clinical utility
α_1-Antitrypsin	Blood	Decreased levels may indicate α_1-antitrypsin deficiency, a cause of liver and lung disease
ApoB-100, APO-B (apolipoprotein B)	Blood	Lipid measurement
aPTT (activated partial thromboplastin time)	Blood	Monitoring of heparin therapy Diagnosis of bleeding disorders
ASMA (anti–smooth muscle antibody)	Blood	Elevated ASMA levels are typically associated with autoimmune hepatitis
ASOT (antistreptolysin O titre)	Blood	Antistreptolysin O indicates recent (weeks to months) infection with group A *Streptococcus*
AST (aspartate transaminase)	Blood	AST is a marker of liver cell damage Note: AST is less specific than ALT
Bilirubin (direct and indirect)		Elevated direct (conjugated) bilirubin: assessment of biliary obstruction Elevated indirect (unconjugated) bilirubin: assessment of hemolysis and liver disease
Bilirubin, total	Blood	Diagnosis and monitoring of hepatobiliary disease
Blood type	Blood	Matching blood for transfusions Assessment of hemolytic disease in newborns
BNP, NT-pro BNP (brain natriuretic peptide, N-terminal prohormone of brain natriuretic peptide)	Blood	Diagnosis and prognosis of heart failure
BUN (blood urea nitrogen)	Blood	Measurement of renal function With creatinine, diagnosis of dehydration
Butyryl ChE (butyrylcholinesterase, also known as pseudocholinesterase)	Blood	Butyryl ChE is elevated in cholinergic toxidromes

Continued on p. 277

Continued from p. 276

Test	Specimen	Clinical utility
c-ANCA (cytoplasmic antineutrophil cytoplasmic antibody)	Blood	c-ANCA is positive in Wegener granulomatosis
C-peptide	Blood	Measurement of endogenous insulin production C-peptide is: • elevated in type 2 diabetes • reduced or absent in type 1 diabetes
CA 125 (cancer antigen 125)	Blood	Tumour marker for monitoring certain types of ovarian cancer
CA 19-9 (cancer antigen 19-9)	Blood	Tumour marker for monitoring certain types of pancreatic cancer
Calcium	Blood	Assessment of bone diseases, certain cancers, hyperparathyroidism, chronic renal disease
Calcium, free or ionized	Blood	Alternative calcium test that may be useful in patients with abnormal serum protein levels
Calprotectin—fecal	Stool	Distinguishing inflammatory bowel disease (positive) from irritable bowel syndrome (negative)
Carboxyhemoglobin	Blood	Assessment of carbon monoxide exposure
Catecholamine	Blood	Diagnosis of pheochromocytoma
CBC (complete blood count)	Blood	Diagnosis of a variety of conditions including infection, anemia, nutritional deficiency, and hematological malignancy
CEA (carcinoembryonic antigen)	Blood	Tumour marker for monitoring colorectal carcinoma
Cell count	Body fluids	Assessment of the number and identity of white blood cells in fluids
Ceruloplasmin	Blood	Diagnosis of Wilson disease
CF (complement fixation)	Blood	Detection of specific antibodies Note: ELISA and PCR have mostly replaced this test

Continued on p. 278

Continued from p. 277

Test	Specimen	Clinical utility
Chloride	Blood	Diagnosis of acid-base, renal, and adrenal disorders
Cholesterol (lipid panel)	Blood	Assessment and monitoring of cardiovascular disease factors
Cholesterol, non-HDL	Blood	Measurement of lipid subclasses other than HDL Note: non-HDL is an alternative target for treatment
Chymotrypsin—fecal	Stool	Diagnosis of chronic pancreatitis
CK (creatine kinase)	Blood	Measurement of muscle injury
CKMB (creatine kinase MB)	Blood	Diagnosis of cardiac injury, specifically myocardial infarction Note: CKMB has been largely replaced by troponin, which is more sensitive
Clostridium difficile antigen detection assay	Stool	Diagnosis of *Clostridium difficile* infection
Clostridium difficile toxin	Stool	Diagnosis of *Clostridium difficile* infection
Closure time	Blood	This test has replaced bleeding time in the diagnosis of qualitative platelet disorders
CMV antibody (cytomegalovirus antibody)	Blood	Diagnosis of CMV infection
CO_2	Blood	Assessment of ventilation and acid base status
Complement	Blood	Monitoring of patients with certain autoimmune disorders
Copper	Blood Urine	Diagnosis of Wilson disease
Cortisol	Blood Saliva Urine	Diagnosis of adrenal disorders
Cortisol, free	24-hour urine collection	Assessment of adrenal disorders

Continued on p. 279

Continued from p. 278

Test	Specimen	Clinical utility
Creatinine	Blood Urine	Assessment of renal function
Creatinine clearance	Blood	Assessment of renal function
CRH stimulation test (corticotropin-releasing hormone stimulation test)	Blood	Differentiation of causes of ACTH-dependent Cushing syndrome Process: this is a provocation test
CRP, hsCRP (C-reactive protein, high sensitivity C-reactive protein)	Blood	CRP: diagnosis of inflammatory disorders and bacterial infection hsCRP: assessment of cardiovascular risk in certain individuals Note: CRP and hsCRP measure the same substance but differ in the sensitivity of the assay; CRP is an acute phase reactant
Cryoglobulin	Blood	Cryoglobulins (immunoglobulins that precipitate at low temperatures) may be associated with lymphoproliferative disorders, infection (notably hepatitis C), and autoimmune disease
Cryoglobulin	Blood	Diagnosis of cryoglobulinemia
Crystal analysis	Joint fluid Urine	Detection and analysis of pathologic crystals (microscopic analysis) Common use: detecting monosodium urate (gout) in joint fluid
Cystine—urine	Urine	Diagnosis of cystinuria
D-dimer	Blood	Diagnosis of deep vein thrombosis and pulmonary embolus
Dexamethasone suppression test	Blood	Differentiation of causes of Cushing syndrome Process: this is a provocation test
DHEA-S (dehydroepiandrosterone sulfate)	Blood	Investigation of adrenal gland function, hirsutism, and precocious puberty
DHT (dihydrotestosterone)	Blood	Assessment of hirsutism, chronic anovulatory syndrome, hypogonadism, and 5α-reductase deficiency

Continued on p. 280

Continued from p. 279

Test	Specimen	Clinical utility
Direct antiglobulin test (Coombs test)	Blood	Detection of antibodies adherent to red blood cells
		Note: the indirect antiglobulin test detects free antibodies in the blood; either direct or indirect may be used in the diagnosis of hemolytic anemia
DNA antibody	Blood	Diagnosis and monitoring of certain autoimmune disorders
DNA probe		Detection of pathogen DNA or specific DNA mutations
		Process: this is a molecular diagnostic technique where labelled short complementary sequences of DNA or RNA (the probe) are hybridized with the sample of interest to determine if the complementary nucleotide sequence is present
Drug screen—urine, comprehensive	Urine	Identification of any drug present
		Process: performed by mass spectrometry (expensive and time-consuming)
Drugs of abuse screen—urine	Urine	Qualitative detection of recent use of several common drugs of abuse, usually including barbiturates, benzodiazepines, cocaine, cannabinoids, opiates, amphetamines, oxycodone, and methadone metabolites
E_2 (estradiol)	Blood	Monitoring of female fertility treatments
E_3 (estriol)	Blood	Prenatal screening
eGFR (estimated glomerular filtration rate)	Blood	Assessment of renal function
		Calculated from serum creatinine by one of several equations
		More sensitive in the detection of early renal disease than creatinine alone

Continued on p. 281

Continued from p. 280

Test	Specimen	Clinical utility
EIA/CIA rapid treponemal-specific immunoassay	Blood	Diagnosis of syphilis
Elastase—fecal	Stool	Assessment of disorders of the exocrine pancreas
Electrolytes—urine	Urine	Assessment of electrolyte and renal disorders
ELISA (enzyme-linked immunosorbent assay)	Blood Other fluids	Detection of antibodies Process: combines surface-bound antibodies with an enzymatic reaction
ENA antibody (extractable nuclear antigen antibody)	Blood	Diagnosis of a number of autoimmune diseases Note: if ENA screen is positive, then follow-up testing is performed for specific antibodies: chromatin, Sm, RNP, SSA-60/Ro, Ro52/TRIM21, SSB/LA, topoisomerase I (Scl-70), Jo-1 (histidyl tRNA synthetase), ribosomal P
Eosinophil count, fecal	Stool	High eosinophil counts are seen in parasitic infections, allergic reactions, and eosinophilic gastroenteritis
EPO (erythropoietin)	Blood	Diagnosis of polycythemia vera (low serum EPO levels is one of the minor criteria)
ESR (erythrocyte sedimentation rate)	Blood	Measurement of inflammation Common use: diagnosis and monitoring of temporal arteritis and polymyalgia rheumatica
Ethylene glycol	Blood	Diagnosis of ethylene glycol poisoning (common component of antifreeze)
Factor V Leiden functional assay	Blood	Investigation of thrombophilia

Continued on p. 282

Continued from p. 281

Test	Specimen	Clinical utility
Fecal occult blood – FIT (fecal immunochemical test) – gFOBT (guaiac fecal occult blood test, being phased out)	Stool	Confirmation of colonic blood loss Common use: screening for colorectal carcinoma Note: • False positives and negatives may occur with FIT or gFOBT, but particularly with gFOBT • gFOBT has false-negative results with vitamin C supplements, and false-positive results with certain foods • FIT detects fecal transferrin, globin, or porphyrin • DNA mutational analysis of stool sample to detect more common cancer-associated genetic mutations is also commercially available, but not in widespread use
Ferritin	Blood	Assessment of iron deficiency anemia
Folate	Blood	Diagnosis of folate deficiency Note: folate deficiency is rare in Canada since universal flour supplementation began several decades ago; it may still be relevant for refugees and new immigrants to Canada
Free light chains (Bence Jones protein)	Urine (24-hour collection or random specimen)	Diagnosis and monitoring of light chain plasma cell dyscrasias
FSH (follicle-stimulating hormone)	Blood	Assessment of ovulation and menopause in females
FTA-ABS (fluorescent treponemal antibody absorption)	Blood	Diagnosis of syphilis
Gentamicin	Blood	Therapeutic monitoring of gentamycin dosing

Continued on p. 283

Continued from p. 282

Test	Specimen	Clinical utility
GGT (γ-glutamyltransferase)	Blood	GGT is a marker of damage to bile duct endothelium
Giardia lamblia cyst antigen assay (ELISA)	Stool	Diagnosis of *Giardia lamblia* infection
Glucose	Blood	Diagnosis and monitoring of diabetes
Glucose—CSF	CSF	Diagnosis of CNS tumour, infection, and inflammation
Glucose, oral tolerance	Blood	Diagnosis of diabetes
Glucose, random or fasting	Blood	Diagnosis of diabetes
Gram stain	Blood Body fluid	Identification of pathologic bacteria
Growth hormone	Blood	Diagnosis of pituitary tumours causing acromegaly (high levels) or growth hormone deficiency and hypopituitarism (low levels)
Haptoglobin	Blood	Haptoglobin is decreased in hemolytic anemia
HbA$_{1c}$ (glycated hemoglobin)	Blood	Diagnosis and monitoring of diabetes
β-hCG—qualitative urine (β-human chorionic gonadotropin)	Urine	Diagnosis of pregnancy
β-hCG—quantitative (β-human chorionic gonadotropin)	Blood	Diagnosis of pregnancy Monitoring of certain malignancies
HDL (high-density lipoprotein)	Blood	Evaluation of cardiovascular risk Note: this is a lipid subclass; higher levels are associated with decreased cardiovascular risk
Hemoglobin electrophoresis	Blood	Diagnosis of hemoglobinopathies
Hemoglobinopathy screen	Blood	Detection of thalassemias, sickle cell disease, and other hemoglobinopathies

Continued on p. 284

Continued from p. 283

Test	Specimen	Clinical utility
Hepatitis (viral) markers	Blood	**Hepatitis A markers** • Hepatitis A IgM antibody is positive in acute infection, IgG positive in chronic infection **Hepatitis B markers** • Negative HBsAg (antigen), anti-HBc (core) and anti-HBs (surface) indicates nonimmune, susceptible individuals • Negative HBsAg, positive anti-HBc, and positive anti-HBs indicates immunity due to naturally acquired infection • Negative HBsAg, negative anti-HBc, and positive anti-HBs indicates immunity due to hepatitis B immunization • Positive HBsAg, positive anti-HBc, and negative anti-HBs indicates active infection; anti-HBc IgM is positive in acute infections and negative in chronic infections • Negative HBsAg, positive anti-HBc, and negative anti-HBs (in combination) may indicate a resolved prior infection or a chronic infection, or may represent a false-positive anti-HBc result • HBeAg (envelope) is generally present in acute infections and the resulting antibody (anti-HBe) appears during convalescence; HBeAg is variably present in chronic infection but may disappear in carriers of the precore HBV mutation **Hepatitis C markers** • Hepatitis C antibody is present in chronic hepatitis C infection
HIV antibody	Blood	Diagnosis of HIV
HLA-B27	Blood	HLA-B27 is usually positive in patients with ankylosing spondylitis
Homocysteine	Blood	Homocysteine is elevated in vitamin B_{12} and folate deficiency Note: this is a controversial cardiovascular risk marker

Continued on p. 285

Continued from p. 284

Test	Specimen	Clinical utility
ICE syphilis recombinant antigen test (immune-capture EIA syphilis recombinant antigen test)		Diagnosis of syphilis
IgA	Blood	Diagnosis of IgA deficiency Monitoring of plasma cell dyscrasias
IgA EMA (IgA antiendomysial antibody)	Blood	Diagnosis of celiac disease
IgA tTGA (IgA tissue transglutaminase antibody)	Blood	Diagnosis of celiac disease
IgG tTGA (IgG transglutaminase antibody)	Blood	Diagnosis of celiac disease in IgA-deficient patients
Immunoglobulins, quantitative	Blood	Assessment of immunodeficiency Monitoring of plasma cell dyscrasias Note: the test includes IgA, IgG and IgM antibodies
Inhibin	Blood	Evaluation of infertility
Insulin	Blood	Assessment of hypoglycemia
Iron	Blood	Assessment of iron deficiency/overload
Ketone screen	Blood	Assessment of ketosis in diabetic or fasting patients Note: this test does not detect acetoacetic acid or acetone
Ketone screen—urine	Random urine	Diagnosis of ketosis, generally in the setting of diabetic ketoacidosis
KOH (potassium hydroxide) scrape prep wet mount evaluation	Skin	Diagnosis of fungal skin or nail infections
Lactate (lactic acid)	Blood	Assessment of acid-base disturbances Prognosis of sepsis
Lactoferrin	Stool	Lactoferrin is increased in active inflammatory bowel disease
LDH (lactate dehydrogenase)	Blood	LDH is elevated in a number of conditions including hemolytic anemia, intestinal and pulmonary infarction, kidney and liver disease, and a number of cancers

Continued on p. 286

Continued from p. 285

Test	Specimen	Clinical utility
LDL (low-density lipoprotein)	Blood	Measurement of lipids Note: LDL is a lipid subclass and a primary target of lipid-lowering medications
Leukocytes—stool	Stool	Leukocytes are elevated in bacterial diarrheal illness
LH (luteinizing hormone)	Blood	Detection of ovulation Assessment of infertility and pituitary disorders
Lipase	Blood	Diagnosis of pancreatitis
Macroprolactin	Blood	Distinguishing true hyperprolactinemia from macroprolactinemia Note: macroprolactinemia should be considered if, in the presence of elevated prolactin levels, signs and symptoms of hyperprolactinemia are absent
Magnesium	Blood	Evaluation of certain electrolyte abnormalities
Metanephrine	24-hour urine collection Blood	Diagnosis of pheochromocytoma
Methanol	Blood	Assessment of methanol poisoning
Methemoglobin	Blood	Diagnosis of methemoglobinemia
MHA-TP (microhemagglutination assay—*Treponema pallidum*)	Blood	Diagnosis of syphilis
Microalbumin (urine albumin)	24-hour urine collection Timed urine collection Random urine specimen	Assessment of proteinuria Common use: monitoring diabetes and chronic renal failure Note: microalbumin is albumin measured at low levels

Continued on p. 287

Continued from p. 286

Test	Specimen	Clinical utility
α_2-Macroglobulin	Blood	Elevated α_2-macroglobulin levels point to nephrotic syndrome
α_1-Microglobulin	Random urine	Assessment of proteinuria
β_2-Microglobulin	Blood	Prognosis of certain blood cancers
Mitochondrial antibody	Blood	Elevated mitochondrial antibody levels are associated with a number of autoimmune conditions
Mixing studies	Blood	Detection of clotting factor deficiencies. Correction of an elevated INR or PTT by mixing 50:50 with normal plasma suggests a factor deficiency, while failure to correct suggests a factor inhibitor
Mono test (heterophile antibody test)	Blood	Diagnosis of infectious mononucleosis Note: this test may take 2 weeks to become positive after onset of symptoms
Mumps serology	Blood	Diagnosis of mumps Note: urine and/or saliva for mumps nucleic acid testing (NAT) is an alternative test
NAAT (nucleic acid amplification testing)	Blood Body fluids	Identification of viruses and bacteria (molecular diagnostic technique)
nRNP (nuclear ribonucleoprotein)	Blood	Antibodies to nRNP are present in most cases of mixed connective tissue disease
Occult blood – *see fecal occult blood*		
OG (osmolal gap)	Blood	Assessment of hypertriglyceridemia, hypergammaglobulinemia, hyperglycemia, and alcohol(s) ingestion *See p. 294 for calculation and other details*

Continued on p. 288

Continued from p. 287

Test	Specimen	Clinical utility
Osmolality	Blood	Diagnosis of poisoning with substances producing an osmolar gap (isopropanol, methanol, ethylene glycol)
		Assessment of ADH (antidiuretic hormone) production
Osmolality—urine	Urine	Increased urine osmolality points to dehydration, SIADH, glycosuria, hypernatremia
		Decreased urine osmolality points to diabetes insipidus, excessive fluid intake, or a renal disorder
Ova and parasites	Stool	Diagnosis of infectious diarrhea
p-ANCA (perinuclear antineutrophil cytoplasmic antibody)	Blood	p-ANCA is positive in ulcerative colitis and other autoimmune diseases
Pap test	Cytology	Detection of cervical dysplasia and malignancy
Parietal cell antibody	Blood	Diagnosis of pernicious anemia
Peripheral blood smear	Blood	Diagnosis of red blood cell, platelet, and white blood cell abnormalities, including leukemia
pH	Blood	Assessment of acid base status
pH—stool	Stool	Acidic stool points to lactose intolerance
Phenytoin (Dilantin)	Blood	Monitoring of phenytoin dosing
Phosphate	Blood	Decreased phosphate concentrations point to hypoparathyroidism, liver disease, and renal failure
		Increased concentrations point to hypercalcemia, hyperparathyroidism, rickets, and osteomalacia
Platelet function assay	Blood	Diagnosis of qualitative abnormalities in platelets
Potassium	Blood	Diagnosis of electrolyte disturbances
Prealbumin (transthyretin)	Blood CSF	Prealbumin is decreased in malnutrition
Prolactin	Blood	Diagnosis of pituitary gland tumours

Continued on p. 289

Continued from p. 288

Test	Specimen	Clinical utility
Protein C and S	Blood	Assessment of hypercoagulable states
Protein—CSF	CSF	CSF protein is elevated in tumours, bleeding, and inflammation
Protein, total	Blood	Total protein is: • decreased in malnutrition and protein-losing diseases • increased in inflammation, infection, multiple myeloma, and Waldenstrom disease
Prothrombin	Blood	Assessment of hypercoagulable states
PSA (prostate-specific antigen)	Blood	Screening for prostate cancer Monitoring of prostate cancer therapy
PSA ratio, free/total (prostate-specific antigen ratio, free/total)	Blood	Diagnosis of prostatic carcinoma Note: • Decreased free/total PSA ratio is associated with a higher incidence of prostatic carcinoma • This test may be useful in determining the need for biopsy in men with mild elevation in PSA
PT/INR (prothrombin time or international normalized ratio)	Blood	Assessment of excessive bleeding and liver function Therapeutic monitoring of warfarin dosing Note: PT and INR are the same test; labs generally report INR and not PT
PTH (parathyroid hormone)	Blood	Investigation of abnormal calcium levels Diagnosis of hyperparathyroidism and hypoparathyroidism
Rapid antigen test	Throat swab	Diagnosis of group A *Streptococcus* pharyngitis
RBC AChE (RBC acetylcholinesterase)	Blood	RBC AChE is elevated in cholinergic toxidromes
Red cell antibody screen	Blood	Detection of anti-RBC antibodies

Continued on p. 290

Continued from p. 289

Test	Specimen	Clinical utility
Renin	Blood	With aldosterone, diagnosis of hyperaldosteronism
Reticulocyte count	Blood	Elevated reticulocyte counts indicate increased red cell production
Reverse T_3 (reverse triiodothyronine)	Blood	No longer recommended
		Previously purported to distinguish nonthyroidal illness from thyroidal illness
RF (rheumatoid factor)	Blood	Diagnosis of rheumatoid arthritis
		Note: RF is commonly elevated in rheumatoid arthritis and other autoimmune diseases, and also in some healthy people, especially older individuals
RPR (rapid plasma reagin)	Blood	Diagnosis of syphilis
Rubella antibody titre	Blood	High levels of rubella antibody indicate immunity to rubella
SAAG (serum-ascites albumin gradient)	Ascites fluid	Assessment of ascites fluid
	Blood	Ascites due to hepatic congestion is associated with an elevated SAAG and a high protein level
		Ascites due to malignancy is associated with a low SAAG and a high protein level
Salicylate	Blood	Assessment and management of salicylate overdose
Sodium	Blood	Diagnosis of electrolyte disturbances
SPE (serum protein electrophoresis)	Blood	Diagnosis and monitoring of plasma cell dyscrasias and other disorders causing abnormal protein concentrations
T_3, free (free triiodothyronine)	Blood	Evaluation of thyroid disorders
		Note: this test is rarely indicated
T_4, free (free thyroxine)	Blood	Evaluation of an elevated TSH result
		A decreased free T_4 points to hypothyroidism

Continued on p. 291

Continued from p. 290

Test	Specimen	Clinical utility
Testosterone, bioavailable	Blood	Evaluation of hypogonadism, infertility, andropause, and osteoporosis
		Note: bioavailable testosterone may be a better indicator of testosterone levels than total and free testosterone
Testosterone, free	Blood	Assessment of male infertility, erectile dysfunction, hirsutism, male osteoporosis
		Monitoring of testosterone-lowering medicines in prostate cancer
Testosterone, total	Blood	Investigation of erectile dysfunction, infertility, testicular tumours, hirsutism, and hypothalamic and pituitary disorders
		Note: testosterone is decreased in male hypogonadism
Thyroglobulin antibodies	Blood	Thyroglobulin antibodies are positive in patients with Hashimoto thyroiditis or Graves disease
TIBC (total iron binding capacity)	Blood	Increased TIBC indicates iron deficiency
		Decreased TIBC indicates iron overload (e.g. hemolytic anemia, hemochromatosis)
TPPA (*Treponema pallidum* particle agglutination)	Blood	Diagnosis of syphilis
Transferrin saturation	Blood	Transferrin saturation values < 20% indicate iron deficiency
		Values > 50% indicate iron overload
Triglyceride	Blood	Diagnosis of hypertriglyceridemia and monitoring of treatment
		Note: triglyceride is a subclass of cholesterol
Troponin	Blood	Diagnosis of cardiac injury, specifically myocardial infarction
TSH (thyroid-stimulating hormone: thyrotropin)	Blood	Diagnosis of hyper- or hypothyroidism

Continued on p. 292

Continued from p. 291

Test	Specimen	Clinical utility
TTKG (transtubular potassium gradient)	Blood	Identifying the etiology of hyper- or hypokalemia
	Urine	*See p. 295 for calculation*
Tzanck smear	Tissue (smear of ulcer base)	Diagnosis of herpes simplex virus (HSV) and varicella zoster virus (VZV)
UPE (urine protein electrophoresis)	24-hour urine collection	Detection of proteins associated with plasma cell dyscrasias (Bence Jones protein, free light chains)
Uric acid (urate)	Blood	Diagnosis and monitoring of gout
Uric acid—urine	Urine	Uric acid is elevated in gout
Urinalysis	Urine	Diagnosis of infection, proteinuria, glycosuria, and hematuria
Varicella antibody	Blood	Elevated values for varicella antibody indicate immunity to varicella
VDRL (Venereal Disease Research Laboratory test)	Blood	Diagnosis of syphilis
Vitamin B_{12}	Blood	Diagnosis of vitamin B_{12} deficiency
Vitamin D (25-hydroxyvitamin D)	Blood	Not recommended as a screening test Low vitamin D levels are associated with certain bone diseases
Vitamin E	Blood	Diagnosis of vitamin E deficiency
Von Willebrand antigen and functional assay (e.g., ristocetin cofactor activity)	Blood	Diagnosis of von Willebrand disease Note: different subtypes of vWF yield different patterns of results
WBC—stool	Stool	WBCs are elevated in inflammatory bowel disease and bacterial diarrhea

Calculations and further information

AG (ANION GAP)

For plasma to remain electrically neutral, the concentration of cations must be equal to that of anions.

The anion gap (AG) describes the excess concentration of measured cations over measured anions.

$$AG = [Na^+] - [Cl^-] - [HCO_3^-]$$

where all units are mmol/L (= mEq/L)

Note that:

- The most commonly measured ions are sodium (Na^+), chloride (Cl^-), bicarbonate (HCO_3^-), and potassium (K^+).
- K^+ is measured, but not typically included in the calculation of AG.
- Some cations are not measured: these commonly include calcium (Ca^{+2}), magnesium (Mg^{+2}), and cationic proteins (primarily IgG).
- Some anions are not measured: anionic proteins such as albumin, and alpha and beta globulins; phosphate (PO_4^{-3}); sulphate (SO_4^{-2}); lactate; and various other acids.

The AG is an insensitive and nonspecific indicator of acidosis. Many factors decrease the AG, which contributes to its insensitivity, including: hypercalcemia; hypermagnesemia; hypoalbuminemia; increased lithium and bromine; and IgG and IgA paraproteinemia.[1]

The reference interval for the AG is approximately 6 to 15 mmol/L (mEq/L). An AG > 20 to 30 mmol/L (mEq/L) is likely clinically significant, signalling metabolic acidosis regardless of the pH and Pco_2.[2(pp48,122)] Note that the AG range is probably the least reproducible and accurate reference interval in the practice of laboratory medicine.[3(p26)]

Increased AGs can have many possible causes (mnemonic: **CAT-MUDPILES**)[2(p49)]:

> **c**arbon monoxide, cyanide, and caffeine
>
> **a**rsenic
>
> **t**oluene
>
> **m**ethanol
>
> **u**remia
>
> **d**iabetic ketoacidosis
>
> **p**araldehyde
>
> **i**ron, isoniazid and ibuprofen
>
> **l**actate and lithium
>
> **e**thanol and ethylene glycol
>
> **s**alicylate and strychnine

Note that almost all increased AGs are due to lactic acidosis, ketoacidosis, and renal failure (uremia).[3(p44)] The next most common cause is intoxication.

OG (OSMOLAL GAP)

The primary molecules that contribute to plasma osmolality are sodium (Na^+), chloride (Cl^-), bicarbonate (HCO_3^-), glucose, and urea.

> Osmolality = $1.86 \times [Na^+] + [glucose] + [urea] + 9$
>
> where osmolality is in mmol/kg ($= mOsm/kg$) and the analytes are in mmol/L ($= mEq/L$)

Reporting of glucose and blood urea nitrogen (BUN) in mg/dL necessitates the introduction of 18 and 2.8 as conversion factors. This yields the following equation:

> Osmolality = $1.86 \times [Na^+] + [glucose]/18 +$ $[BUN]/2.8 + 9$

The osmolal gap is the difference between the osmolality measured by freezing point depression and that predicted by the equation.

A typical reference interval for OG is < 10 mmol/kg (mOsm/kg).

The more common causative agents for an elevated measured osmolality with a normal calculated osmolality include (mnemonic: **ME DIE**):

>**m**ethanol
>
>**e**thanol
>
>**d**iuretics (mannitol, sorbitol, glycerol)
>
>**i**sopropanol
>
>**e**thylene glycol

Other possible intoxicants include acetone, chloroform, diethyl ether, isoniazid, paraldehyde, and trichloroethane.

TTKG (TRANSTUBULAR POTASSIUM GRADIENT)

Calculate TTKG as follows:

$$\text{TTKG} = \frac{\text{urine}_{K+}}{\text{plasma}_{K+}} \div \frac{\text{urine}_{osm}}{\text{plasma}_{osm}}$$

REFERENCES

1 Charney AN, Hoffman RS. Fluid, electrolyte, and acid-base principles. In: Flomenbaum NE, Howland MA, Goldfrank LR, Lewin NA, Hoffman RS, Lewis SN, eds. *Goldfrank's Toxicologic Emergencies.* 8th ed. New York, NY: McGraw-Hill; 2006:278–295.

2 Ellenhorn MJ. *Ellenhorn's Medical Toxicology: Diagnosis and Treatment of Human Poisoning.* 2nd ed. Baltimore, MD: Williams and Wilkins; 1997.

3 Alter D, Dufour DR. Anion gap: a review. ASCP teleconference [transcript]. American Society for Clinical Pathology. October 17, 2012.

Abbreviations

6-AM	6-monoacetylmorphine	ChE	cholinesterase
ABG	arterial blood gas	CHF	congestive heart failure
ACh	acetylcholine	CK	creatine kinase
AChE	acetylcholinesterase	CKMB	creatine kinase MB
AChR	acetylcholine receptor	CML	chronic myelocytic leukemia
AChR antibody	acetylcholine receptor antibody	CMML	chronic myelomonocytic leukemia
		CMV	cytomegalovirus
ACTH	adrenocorticotropic hormone	CNS	central nervous system
ADH	antidiuretic hormone	COPD	chronic obstructive pulmonary disease
AFP	α$_1$-fetoprotein		
AG	anion gap	CRF	chronic renal failure
ALC-1	anti–liver cytosol antibody type 1	CRH	corticotropin-releasing hormone
ALKM-1	anti–liver kidney microsomal antibody type 1	CRP	C-reactive protein
		CSF	cerebrospinal fluid
ALP	alkaline phosphatase	CT	computed tomography
ALT	alanine aminotransferase	CYP2E1	cytochrome P450 2E1
AMA	antimitochondrial antibodies	DAT	direct antiglobulin test
ANA	antinuclear antibodies	DFA	direct fluorescence assay
anti-CCP	cyclic citrullinated polypeptide antibody	DHEA-S	dehydroepiandrosterone-sulfate
		DI	diabetes insipidus
anti-TPO	anti–thyroid peroxidase	DIC	disseminated intravascular coagulation
APO-B	apolipoprotein B		
aPTT	activated partial thromboplastin time	DKA	diabetic ketoacidosis
		DNA	deoxyribonucleic acid
ARF	acute renal failure	DRE	digital rectal exam
ASA	acetylsalicylic acid	DVT	deep vein thrombosis
ASMA	anti–smooth muscle antibody	E$_2$	estradiol
AST	aspartate aminotransferase	E$_3$	estriol
AT	antithrombin	EBV	Epstein-Barr virus
ATP	adenosine triphosphate	ECG	electrocardiogram
AV	atrioventricular	EDTA	ethylenediaminetetraacetic acid
BMI	body-mass index	EGD	esophagogastroduodenoscopy
BP	blood pressure	eGFR	estimated glomerular filtration rate
BPH	benign prostatic hyperplasia	EIA	enzyme immunoassay
BUN	blood urea nitrogen	ELISA	enzyme-linked immunosorbent assay
CA 125	cancer antigen 125		
CA 19-9	cancer antigen 19-9	EMA	antiendomysial antibody
CBC	complete blood count	ENA	extractable nuclear antigen
CEA	carcinoembryonic antigen	EPO	erythropoietin

ERCP	endoscopic retrograde cholangiopancreatography
ESR	erythrocyte sedimentation rate
FIT	fecal immunochemical test
FNA	fine needle aspiration
FPG	fasting plasma glucose
FSH	follicle-stimulating hormone
FTA-ABS	fluorescent treponemal antibody absorption test
G6PD	glucose-6-phosphate dehydrogenase deficiency
GABA	γ-aminobutyric acid
GBM	glomerular basement membrane
GBS	group B *Streptococcus*
GERD	gastroesophageal reflux disease
gFOBT	guaiac fecal occult blood test
GFR	glomerular filtration rate
GGT	γ-glutamyltransferase
GI	gastrointestinal
GU	genitourinary
HAV	hepatitis A virus
Hb	hemoglobin
HbA$_{1c}$	glycated hemoglobin
HBcAb	hepatitis B core antibody
HBeAb	hepatitis B e antibody
HBsAb	hepatitis B surface antibody
HBsAg	hepatitis B surface antigen
HBV	hepatitis B virus
hCG	human chorionic gonadotropin
Hct	hematocrit
HCV	hepatitis C virus
HDL	high-density lipoprotein
HELLP	**h**emolysis, **el**evated liver enzymes, **l**ow **p**latelet count
HEV	hepatitis E virus
HHS	hyperosmolar hyperglycemic state
HIT	heparin-induced thrombocytopenia
HIV	human immunodeficiency virus
HPF	high power microscopic field
HPV	human papillomavirus
hsCRP	high sensitivity C-reactive protein
HSV	herpes simplex virus
HUS	hemolytic uremic syndrome
IBD	inflammatory bowel disease
ICE	immune-capture EIA
IFA	immunofluorescent assay
IFT	impaired fasting glucose
IgA	immunoglobulin A
IgG	immunoglobulin G

IgM	immunoglobulin M
IGT	impaired glucose tolerance
IM	intramuscular
INR	international normalized ratio
ITP	immune thrombocytopenia
IV	intravenous
IVC	inferior vena cava
KOH	potassium hydroxide
KUB	kidneys, ureter, bladder X-ray
LCR	ligase chain reaction
LDH	lactate dehydrogenase
LDL	low-density lipoprotein
LDL-C	low-density lipoprotein cholesterol
LE	leukocyte esterase
LFT	liver function test
LH	luteinizing hormone
LOC	level of consciousness
LSD	lysergic acid diethylamide
MAHA	microangiopathic hemolytic anemia
MAOI	monoamine oxidase inhibitor
MCH	mean corpuscular hemoglobin
MCHC	mean corpuscular hemoglobin concentration
MCV	mean corpuscular volume
MDA	3,4-methylenedioxyamphetamine
MDMA	3,4-methylenedioxy-*N*-methylamphetamine
MGUS	monoclonal gammopathy
MHA-TP	microhemagglutination assay–*Treponema pallidum*
MMDA	3-methoxy-4,5-methylenedioxyamphetamine
MMR	measles-mumps-rubella vaccine
MRI	magnetic resonance imaging
MRSA	methicillin-resistant *Staphylococcus aureus*
NAAT	nucleic acid amplification testing
NAPQI	N-acetylbenzoquinoneimine
NGSP	National Glycohemoglobin Standardization Program
NSAID	nonsteroidal anti-inflammatory drug
NT	nuchal translucency
NT-pro BNP	N-terminal prohormone of brain natriuretic peptide
O+P	ova and parasites
OCP	oral contraceptive
OG	osmolality gap
OGTT	oral glucose tolerance test

p-ANCA	perinuclear antineutrophil cytoplasmic antibody	SNRI	serotonin/norepinephrine reuptake inhibitor
PAPP-A	pregnancy-associated plasma protein A	SPE	serum protein electrophoresis
PBC	primary biliary cirrhosis	SSRI	selective serotonin reuptake inhibitor
PCOS	polycystic ovary syndrome	SSSS	staphylococcal scalded skin syndrome
PCP	phencyclidine		
PCR	polymerase chain reaction	STD	sexually transmitted disease
PE	pulmonary embolism	T_3	triiodothyronine
PK	pharmacokinetics	T_4	thyroxine
po	orally	TB	tuberculosis
PSA	prostate-specific antigen	TCA	tricyclic antidepressant
PSC	primary sclerosing cholangitis	TDM	therapeutic drug monitoring
PT	prothrombin time	THC	tetrahydrocannabinol
PT/INR	prothrombin time or international normalized ratio	TIA	transient ischemic attack
		TIBC	total iron binding capacity
PTH	parathyroid hormone	TPO	thyroid peroxidase
PTT	partial thromboplastin time	TPPA	*Treponema pallidum* particle agglutination
RAST	radioallergosorbent test		
RBC	red blood cell	TRH	thyrotropin-releasing hormone
RDW	red blood cell distribution width	TSH	thyroid-stimulating hormone (thyrotropin)
RF	rheumatoid factor		
RPR	rapid plasma reagin	tTG	tissue transglutaminase
RR	respiration rate	TTKG	transtubular potassium gradient
RT-PCR	reverse transcription polymerase chain reaction	TTP	thrombotic thrombocytopenic purpura
RTA	renal tubular acidosis	UTI	urinary tract infection
SAAG	serum-ascites albumin gradient	VDRL	Venereal Disease Research Laboratory test
SIADH	syndrome of inappropriate antidiuretic hormone secretion		
		VTE	venous thromboembolism
SLE	systemic lupus erythematosus	vWF	von Willebrand factor
		WBC	white blood cell

Contributors

Dr. Leland B. Baskin is a general pathologist. He is Medical Director and Vice President for Medical Operations at Calgary Laboratory Services, and a clinical associate professor in the Department of Pathology and Laboratory Medicine at the University of Calgary.

Dr. Launny Faulkner is a general pathology resident at the University of Calgary. She studied zoology at the University of Victoria and is a graduate of the University of British Columbia Island Medical Program.

Dr. Ethan Flynn is a general pathologist with extensive teaching and administrative experience. He is an associate professor in the Department of Pathology and Laboratory Medicine at the University of Calgary, and General Pathologist and Medical Lead, General Pathology, South Health Campus, Calgary Laboratory Services.

Dr. Christopher Naugler is a general pathologist and family physician with wide-ranging research, teaching, and clinical experience. He is an associate professor in the Department of Pathology and Laboratory Medicine, and the Department of Family Medicine, at the University of Calgary, and Clinical Section Chief of General Pathology with Calgary Laboratory Services.

Dr. Davinder Sidhu is a senior resident in general pathology at the University of Calgary. He is extensively involved in both undergraduate and postgraduate medical education, and has interests in several fields of research. In addition to his medical training (MD), he has degrees in in pharmacy (B.Pharm) and law (LLB).

Index